SpringerBriefs in Psychology

SpringerBriefs present concise summaries of cutting-edge research and practical applications across a wide spectrum of fields. Featuring compact volumes of 50 to 125 pages, the series covers a range of content from professional to academic. Typical topics might include:

- A timely report of state-of-the-art analytical techniques
- A bridge between new research results as published in journal articles and a contextual literature review
- A snapshot of a hot or emerging topic
- An in-depth case study or clinical example
- A presentation of core concepts that readers must understand to make independent contributions

SpringerBriefs in Psychology showcase emerging theory, empirical research, and practical application in a wide variety of topics in psychology and related fields. Briefs are characterized by fast, global electronic dissemination, standard publishing contracts, standardized manuscript preparation and formatting guidelines, and expedited production schedules.

More information about this series at http://www.springer.com/series/10143

Martin M. Katz

Clinical Trials of Antidepressants

How Changing the Model Can Uncover New, More Effective Molecules

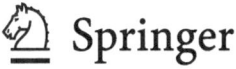 Springer

Martin M. Katz
Health Science Center at San Antonio
University of Texas
San Antonio, TX
USA

ISSN 2192-8363   ISSN 2192-8371   (electronic)
SpringerBriefs in Psychology
ISBN 978-3-319-26463-9   ISBN 978-3-319-26464-6   (eBook)
DOI 10.1007/978-3-319-26464-6

Library of Congress Control Number: 2015958328

Printed on acid-free paper

This Springer imprint is published by SpringerNature
The registered company is Springer International Publishing AG Switzerland

Foreword

In this timely, succinct book, Dr. Katz explains the clinical trial methodology required by the FDA for putative antidepressants for half a century. The resultant studies have been effective in determining whether a new drug is significantly more effective than a placebo in a double-blind trial of several weeks. However, the design does nothing to elucidate the mechanism of action of the drug molecule, nor which symptom components are benefitted, which are unaffected and whether any components are worsened. The approach he recommends aims to provide a profile of the drug's clinical actions on discrete components, e.g., insomnia, slowed movements, as well as the sequence and timing of such actions.

Katz takes the reader through the aims of traditional disorder-specific trials, in particular the consequences of selecting a scale such as the Hamilton Depression Rating Scale (Ham-D) total score as the outcome measure. The Ham-D does well enough in estimating time of onset of clinical action, but not the symptom dimensions, also called domains, that comprise major depression. Therefore, the very aims that could identify differences between treatments on the timing, sequence, or domain profile of the disorder are beyond the capabilities of the method. An example is the relationship of a drug's impact on a particular neurotransmitter system, e.g., norepinephrine; and the specific behaviors understood to be functionally linked to noradrenergic activity. The component-specific model he supports provides information on the nature of drug-induced clinical actions, as well as onset and sequence of effect.

He summarizes recent and older studies which consistently indicate that a large proportion of antidepressant drugs' benefits occur within the first 3 weeks of treatment. Katz has been a pioneer of studies addressing analysis of early actions of antidepressants on specific behavioral, symptomatic components of depression. He summarizes how the fine-grained results obtained from employing component-enriched depression rating scales concomitantly with video taping can support important advances in both treatments and neurobiology of depression. The enhanced sensitivity of the video method over the Ham-D in picking up discrete behavioral components is partly consequent to the video-based method's sensitivity to measuring physically expressive and social behaviors, rather than just reported components of depression.

Katz writes briefly about the nature of FDA review of submitted clinical trials. "It appears that once one gets beyond the optimal dosage and marketability issues, there is no further use to which the study can be put. The reason is that it is known from prior studies that the Ham-D cannot provide reliable information on any of the aspects or components of major depressive disorder." He closes with what I believe to be an important observation. "If the treatment turned out to be non-efficacious for that disorder, the study could, by way of an analysis of the nature and sequence of changes brought about by the agent, provide a profile of information on behavioral and neurochemical changes which could advance understanding of the target disorder or the neurobehavioral mechanisms underlying the efficacy or non-efficacy of the new treatment agent. No longer an exercise in applied research, the clinical trial becomes a potential step in facilitating the advance to finding new and more effective treatments for this major mental disorder."

Charles L. Bowden, M.D.
Clinical Professor of Psychiatry and Pharmacology
Nancy U. Karren
Endowed Professor of Psychiatry
University of Texas, Health Science Center San Antonio

Preface

The current conduct of clinical trials of new antidepressants is based on a model developed five decades earlier and now turns out to be very wasteful. Too many drugs with unusual, potentially therapeutic actions have been found to be non-efficacious. It appears to be due in great part to the methodology used in such trials to evaluate efficacy. The established model utilizes only the Hamilton Rating Scale for Depression (Ham-D) (1960), an instrument valid for measuring severity of the overall disorder but insensitive to the measurement of change in major components of depression. Viewing the established trial as it is conducted today, we learn whether a new drug significantly reduces the severity of the overall disorder, but gains little to no knowledge about its onset and its profile of clinical actions. Consequently, clinical trials have added little to the advance of science in clinical psychopharmacology. This has lagged the development of new, more effective drugs and waning interest among the pharmaceutical companies to continue active research and drug development in this sphere.

In the interest of overcoming these handicaps and advancing the field, this book puts forth new models for conducting clinical trials. The new models take advantage of knowledge gained over the past five decades on the nature of the depressive disorders. It emphasizes the concept of dimensionality, and new findings on the neurobehavioral mechanisms underlying the efficacy of antidepressant drugs. I trust that such new analyses will bring clinical trials closer to the world of science, and help in moving the field in equally new directions.

Acknowledgments

I attribute my awakening in this field of neurobehavioral research first, to the late James W. Maas who led our initial major effort in 1970 into collaborative research on the psychobiology of depression. I have since continued to work over the long term with Charles L. Bowden and Alan Frazer at the University of Texas Health Science Center at San Antonio who have been steadfast in helping to uncover new findings on the nature of the disorder and the patterns of drug-induced clinical actions. The research has also depended greatly on sound guidance and application of the most appropriate statistics to test the several important hypotheses generated from the early work. For that guidance and collaboration, I thank Nancy Berman whose expertise shows clearly throughout the book.

My daughter, Nancie Katz-Kirtchuk, an investigative journalist, and my son, Pete Katz, a broadcast journalist, assisted greatly in the editing of the final manuscript.

Finally, I wish to thank my wife, Barbara, for her early reading, and patience in helping to see this effort to a hopefully, successful conclusion.

Martin M. Katz

Contents

1 Introduction   1

2 Why Now the Need for a New Clinical Trials Model
   for Antidepressants?   5

3 Reconceptualizing Depression, and the Current Scene
   on Dimensionality and the RDoC   9
   "Opposed Neurobehavioral States"   11
   On Replacing Diagnosis with Dimensions: The Current
   Scene and the RDoC   12

4 Aims and Basic Requirements of Clinical Trials: Conventional
   and Component-Specific Models   13

5 Methods for Measuring the Components and the Profile
   of Drug Actions: The Multivantaged Approach   17

6 Achieving the "Ideal" Clinical Trial: An Example of Applying
   the Merged Componential and Established Models   21
   Applying the Models   22
   Measurement of Behavioral Components and Severity
   of Depressed State   23

7 Comparing the Component-Specific Model Directly
   with the Established Diagnosis-Specific Trial   27
   Secondary Aims   27

8 Prediction and Shortening the Clinical Trial: Further
   Advantages of the Component-Specific Model   31

9 The Video Clinical Trial   35
   Special Application in Multicenter Trials and Proof-of-Concept Studies . . .   37

10 Conclusions   39

**Appendix I: Four Case Studies of Patients in Multivantage (MV) and
  Video Models of Clinical Trials: Instructions for Scoring MV
  Components and Dimensions and Video Measure Profiles....   41**

**Appendix II: Operational Definitions of State Constructs
  and Global Outcome Measures.......................   51**

**Appendix III: Composition and Scoring of Constructs,
  Dimensions and Overall Severity Measures.............   53**

**Appendix IV: MV Methods for Measuring Constructs
  and Outcome Dimensions, Brief Version
  for Outpatient Studies 59**

References   61

Index..   65

List of Figures

Figure 3.1   Depressive disorders and normal controls: baseline
patterns of behavioral and affect constructs. Reproduced
with permission of publisher from Katz et al. (1984).
© Psychological Reports 1984   10

Figure 5.1   *Early drug actions*: comparing treatments across time
periods on hostility. DMI and paroxetine reduce hostility
at a significantly faster rate during the first 2 weeks than
placebo (slopes test $p < 0.05$). At day 13 of treatment
DMI improved hostility significantly more than placebo
*$p < 0.05$, ANCOVA). Reproduced with permission
of publisher from Katz et al. (2004)
Neuropsychopharmacology   18

Figure 5.2   *Early drug actions*: comparing DMI, paroxetine, and placebo
across time periods. **a** *Motor retardation*: at days 7 and 13
of treatment DMI improved motor retardation significantly
more than that caused by either paroxetine or placebo
(**$p < 0.01$, ANCOVA) and at day 10, the same effect
was observed (*$p < 0.05$, ANCOVA). **b** *Severity dimension*:
DM-MR at days 7 and 13 of treatment DMI improved the
severity dimension significantly more than that due to either
paroxetine or placebo (**$p < 0.01$, ANCOVA) and at day
10, the improvement caused by DMI was significantly
greater than that caused by paroxetine (*$p < 0.05$, ANCOVA).
Although behavioral assessments were conducted at
days 21, 28, and 35 of treatment these time points were
not essential for the hypothesis being tested. Consequently,
values obtained at these time points are omitted from
Figs. 3.1a, b and 5.1 for the clarity of data presentation.
Reproduced with permission of publisher from Katz et al.
(2004) Neuropsychopharmacology   19

List of Tables

Table 4.1   Models for design of antidepressant trials:
disorder-specific versus component-specific   14

Table 5.1   Assumptions that guided early trials versus
evidence-based findings   18

Table 7.1   Time of onset of improvement in treatment responders
(survival analysis)...................................   28

Table 7.2   Results from applying componential approach compared
with established diagnosis-specific trial...................   29

Table 9.1   Advantages of video trials   36

Table 9.2   Brief VIBES factors and severity dimensions   36

Chapter 1
Introduction

Today we note that successive failures of clinical trials for new, putative antide-pressants have led pharmaceutical companies to virtually abandon new drug devel-opment in this sphere. Recent events have highlighted the weaknesses and expense of the conventional trial, a model for evaluating new treatments developed more than 50 years ago. There is much agreement that a new model is necessary to res-timulate research interest and activity in this sphere.

Currently when a new drug in a clinical trial is found to be ineffective in sig-nificantly reducing the severity of the targeted disorder, little to no information is recorded on its clinical actions other than that. There is no further evaluation for example as to the drugs' possible effects on various behavioral, mood, or cognitive facets of the disorder. This gap is due to the lack of any methods directly used in the trial, to evaluate such aspects. A case in point is the antidepressant trial, where the sole measuring instrument for the drug's potential behavioral actions, is the Hamilton Depression Rating Scale. This method is valid for measuring changes in the severity of the overall disorder, but is not reliable or valid for measuring changes in key facets of that disorder (e.g., Gibbons et al. 1993).

Information on behavioral changes exist for drugs that are found in clinical trials to be efficacious for the targeted disorder, but not those which are not effi-cacious. If this information did exist, then an important background of findings would be developed to assist in advancing science in this area. The information required tracks the changes that are observed first in central monoaminergic sys-tems that presumably, identify the new drug as potentially effective for this dis-order. Secondly, it links these changes to changes in specific behavioral, mood or cognitive aspects of the disorder. If such findings on drugs in these hundreds of studies were forthcoming, a network of background information would be assem-bled. This network would then be analyzed for uncovering associations between changes in the specific central neurotransmitter systems with changes in the basic behavioral and mood and cognitive factors associated with the disorder. This data

© The Author(s) 2016   1
M.M. Katz, *Clinical Trials of Antidepressants*, SpringerBriefs in Psychology,
DOI 10.1007/978-3-319-26464-6_1

has obvious advantages at all levels of the development process, primarily for the science of clinical psychopharmacology. But more specifically, it can be expected to enhance thinking about developments in neurochemistry and how to design agents with novel targets. The targets might possibly be critical behavioral and emotional aspects of each of the various mental disorders.

At the clinical or practical level, this approach also makes it more possible to identify more potentially effective or more rapidly acting treatments for a range of disorders. Some drugs which have been found to be non-efficacious for a targeted disorder or failed in a clinical trial may—because of unexpected actions on other important aspects of the targeted syndrome—turn out to be effective in the treatment of other mental disorders. One example would be the follow-up discovery regarding trials on *that a major action of the* selective serotonergic reuptake inhibitors (SSRIs). Its specificity in reducing anxiety was in great part responsible for its efficacy for the targeted depressive disorders, *was its specificity in reducing anxiety* (e.g., Dunbar and Fuell 1992). Anxiety, a significant component of the depressive disorders, is also a major component of psychopathology, generally, which in turn is central to many other of the mental disorders. Specifically, it is central for the "anxiety states". The SSRIs were not only found to be effective for anxiety. It turned out that they were more effective for the "generalized" subtype of this disorder than the then established treatment, the benzodiazepines (Kahn et al. 1989).

The conventional trial is designed to provide an either-or decision about a putative treatment drug, essentially applying a simple randomized controlled trial research design to answer an efficacy question. The trial itself as applied science is sound; it includes the required characteristics of a controlled study design, that is, selection of validly diagnosed patients, randomization of patients to the experimental drug or placebo control, appropriate time points for measuring change and "double-blind" conditions for ratings by clinical observers, to evaluate change. Where the conventional trial is deficient from a scientific viewpoint, is in its method of evaluating change. As in the case of the antidepressant trial it relies solely on one measure of change, the Hamilton symptom rating scale (1960) or the similar Montgomery-Asberg Depression Rating scale (MADRS) (1979). These methods as noted, are demonstrably valid for measuring change in overall severity. However, they unreliable and invalid for measuring the major behavioral, mood, or cognitive opponents of the disorder. The result is that conclusions drawn from such studies are confined to indicating whether the experimental drug was or was not significantly more effective than the placebo in reducing the severity of the targeted disorder.

From a scientific and from a practical laboratory viewpoint, this is very little information to reap from this highly expensive clinical trial. It provides paltry new information capable of being used to advance the science in this area, or to enhance the process of new drug development. In fact, the conventional trials model turns out to be wasteful regarding the neurochemical mechanisms associated with its therapeutic actions and the specific actions on the psychological aspects of the disorders *the conventional trials model turns out to be a wasteful procedure.* There is every reason to devote great attention to how detailed and precise information on the actions of a promising, new carefully, developed treatment drugs is generated. The scientific viewpoint on background of information that details on the one hand, the neurochemical changes affected by the drug and on the other, their possible associations with drug-induced behavioral changes, provides a network that can lead to advances in the applications of the treatment. It can potentially, e.g., be applied to treat disorders other than the targeted one. Such disorders would have prominent behavioral components, which the clinical trial would identify.

It is not as if the field has not been aware of the deficiencies of the clinical trial. There has been much effort among clinical investigators to improve on procedures. Notably, there have been attempts to make the Hamilton more efficient and effective in carrying out its role (e.g., Bech 2011) and improvements in the statistics designed to test more sensitively the differences between treatment groups (e.g., Kraemer 2013) and even to introduce more detailed versions of the approach to observational ratings (Rush et al. 1986). Acknowledging that the conventional trial is a sound procedure for determining the efficacy of a new, putative antidepressant, it is by its nature, an expensive effort. The attempts to further refine the Hamilton Scale and to sharpen the statistical approaches to achieving greater sensitivity are to be lauded. However, again, minimal attention has been directed to the most critical aspect of the clinical trial, broadening and intensifying the analysis of the clinical and behavioral changes brought about by the new agents.

Here, I propose to shift the focus on evaluation to measuring with more precision the elemental changes in the behavior, mood and cognitive components of the depressive disorders. The aim is a more precise analysis of what the drug actually accomplishes in its actions on the patient's clinical state. This model's more detailed nature may appear to be even more expensive than the conventional trial. However, it is markedly less costly because it is significantly more scientifically informative for clinical trials of antidepressants. Further, its efficiency shows greater attention to early changes. It will also—as I will describe in a later chapter—make it possible to shorten the trial, a modification that will have important cost, clinical and research implications.

The new model is described in the next chapter.

Chapter 2
Why Now the Need for a New Clinical Trials Model for Antidepressants?

What have we learned during the past 5 decades that makes the established model appear to be out of date, too expensive and based on the wrong principles? If we review the theoretical context upon which the original model was based we recall that it drew its strength from the following assumptions held at that time about how the drugs, in this case the revolutionary antidepressants, actually worked, that is, the neurochemical bases of their efficacy.

These assumptions were as follows: (1) Imipramine due to its capacity to inhibit the reuptake of monoamine neurotransmitters, norepinephrine and serotonin, results in higher levels of these neurotransmitters made available in the synapses of the nervous system. (2) It may not have been shown that these neurotransmitter concentrations are significantly lower in the depressive disorders than in healthy controls. However, it is clear that increasing the availability of these neurotransmitters, as occurs with the administration of the tri-cyclic antidepressants, results in significant improvement *of the disorder*. (3) It therefore, appears that the tri-cyclic antidepressants are specific as treatments for the major depressive disorders. (4) Kuhn in his original report on the efficacy of imipramine (1959) also noted that some patients responded quickly, within the 1st week. The general rule for the majority of patients, however, was to require several weeks to achieve remission of clinical symptoms.

Thus, it was generally accepted that the tri-cyclic antidepressants were in fact, "antidepressants", meaning treatments specific for the diagnosis of major depressive disorder. Despite the almost immediate effects on monoamine neurotransmitters, however, the usual course for the patient responder was not to achieve full clinical response, until several weeks of treatment.

The established clinical trial for evaluating new putative "antidepressants" was designed in accordance with these assumptions. Thus, the trial would extend over 4–12 weeks. The patient sample would consist of diagnosed major depressive disorders; the major assessment points for measuring change would be at baseline and

© The Author(s) 2016   5
M.M. Katz, *Clinical Trials of Antidepressants*, SpringerBriefs in Psychology,
DOI 10.1007/978-3-319-26464-6_2

outcome (since clinical effects, were not expected for several weeks). The major instrument for evaluating change would be a scale of overall severity of the diagnosed disorder. That model has been applied in the hundreds (possibly thousands) of clinical trials since the discovery of imipramine in 1959. It has been a generally effective model for identifying efficacious treatments, including the more recently developed selective serotonin re-uptake inhibitors (SSRIs) (Wong et al. 1974).

During the course of these 50 years, there have been many attempts to improve components of the model. As noted, statistical analyses were refined, and the efficiency or sensitivity of the Hamilton rating scale was improved. A scale focused on measuring change, for example, the Montgomery-Asberg Depression Rating Scale (MADRS) (1979), was introduced. However, there have been no substantive changes in the model, which viewed the target of treatment as the diagnosed disorder. That approach only noted the important change in severity as not occurring for several weeks, and focused exclusively on change of overall severity *of the disorder* as the measure of the efficacy of treatment.

There was in other words, no attention to the not-so-subtle changes in the understanding of how the drugs work and the nature of the clinical condition as these concepts have evolved based on new research during these past 5 decades. It is useful at this point to revisit questions and to review some of the more recent findings that introduce new information and have had some impact on how we develop and then evaluate new treatment agents for these disorders. For example:

1. Are established agents, the tricyclic antidepressants (TCAs) and SSRIs, specific for the treatment of diagnosed depressions?

Basic investigations of the mechanisms of neurobehavioral actions of TCAs and the SSRIs since then have painted a more refined picture of their actions. It has been determined that drug-induced change in the concentration of the norepinephrine metabolite, MHPG, is associated specifically, for example, with motor activity, changes in the serotonin metabolite, 5-HIAA, with anxiety and impulsive hostility. These changes in concentration are not therefore, associated specifically with a diagnosed disorder, but their actions explained more parsimoniously, as associated with the components of the disorder, that is, with behaviors, mood, and/ or cognition. We found in our own research (Katz et al. 1994) such specific associations when treating depression in the studies in psychobiology (Maas et al. 1980).

2. Do clinical actions begin within the 1st 2 weeks, sometimes within the 1st week of treatment?

Research from 1987 on has established this. A series of independent and several multisite, large patient sample studies (Katz et al. 1987; Stassen et al. 1993; Machado et al. 2008; Szegedi et al. 2009) have shown that the major part of the clinical response to the drugs occurs within the 1st 2 weeks. In fact, 70 % of the total response occurs during the 1st 3 weeks (Stassen et al. 1997, 2007); 70 % of patients who show this early improvement go on to achieve a full response; less than 10 % of patients who do not show this early improvement, do not respond at outcome to the drug (Posternak and Zimmerman 2005; Taylor et al. 2006).

It is clear that serious assessment of clinical changes must begin at one week of treatment and be assessed weekly throughout the treatment period.

3. Changes brought about on behavioral components of the disorder are shown to begin as early as 1 week. That supports the judgment that the mechanisms that lead to full clinical response, are initiated by the effects on neurotransmitters. Those neurochemical effects have been found in turn, to be associated differentially with specific behaviors, mood or and cognition, not directly with "whole disorders" (Morilak and Frazer 2004).

These findings do not fully explain the bases for the efficacy of the tri-cyclic antidepressants and the SSRI's in resolving depression, but they do extend understanding of the neurobehavioral mechanisms underlying their efficacy.

It can be shown that the increased availability of serotonin results in reductions in anxiety and anger in the patient, and that increased norepinephrine reduces motor retardation and relieves depressed mood. These, potential changes in the disorder of the patient appeared to evolve into resolving the disorder as a whole (see Delgado (2000) for evidence that confirms the specific therapeutic roles of serotonin and norepinephrine). It is also true that despite all of these advances in understanding, there are still no "biological markers" for the depressive disorders.

Nevertheless we are today in a more advanced stage of understanding how these drugs work, than we were 5 decades ago. These new findings should affect how we develop and how we evaluate new agents for the depressive disorder.

To summarize, the following findings should contribute to modifying how we design a clinical trial: (1) the neurotransmitter systems most impacted by the TCAs and SSRIs are apparently responsible for the changes in the disorder, and (2) the noradrenergic and serotonergic systems are associated with the regulation of different patterns of mood and behavioral components of the disorders. They are not shown to be associated specifically, with the "whole" diagnosed disorder. The focus on assessing changes in the disorder in any new trial should be on the new drugs' impact on these components, as well as on changes in the severity of the overall disorder. That means in practical terms that the methods of evaluation of drug clinical actions should include, but go beyond that measured by the Hamilton or MADRS scales, i.e., methods should be added that are designed to measure the major behavioral, mood and cognitive components.

1. Contrary to earlier notions that nothing of clinical importance changes during the 1st few weeks of treatment, it is very clear that when the drug is effective for treating a targeted disorder, that not only does early improvement appear but that its presence or absence, is predictive of the type of response, positive or negative, to occur at outcome of treatment. Therefore, assessment must begin early, preferably by the end of the first week and then be conducted on a weekly basis throughout the course of treatment. Further, since it has been established that such early changes that may occur may more likely be on components rather than simply on severity of the whole disorder, behavioral methods for the measurement of these behavioral componential changes should be part of the assessment battery.

2. It has also been found that drugs that have specific actions on dimensions of psychopathology, such as anxiety-agitation, dimensions that are critical parts of other mental disorders, like generalized anxiety or obsessive-compulsive disorders, may, although found to be ineffective for the targeted disorder, such as depression, be applicable to the treatment of other allied conditions (for example, as noted the SSRIs are now the preferred treatment for generalized anxiety disorders). Therefore, it is essential to both determine, whether the experimental drug is effective or ineffective for the targeted disorder and the drug's profile of clinical actions on the components of the disorder. The latter assures that this potentially very important information is not lost or neglected, markedly limiting the overall value of this highly expensive clinical trial. It is also necessary to test whether early improvement appears, and be aware that its presence or absence is predictive of the type of clinical response, positive or negative, that will occur at outcome of treatment. Therefore assessment of change must begin early and be conducted sequentially, starting preferably at the end of the 1st week and then conducted regularly on a weekly basis throughout the course of treatment. Further, since it has been established that such early changes that may occur will more likely be on components, rather than simply on overall severity of the disorder, behavioral methods for the measurement of these componential changes should be part of the assessment battery.

These facts accumulated over the past five decades, the results of basic and clinical investigations of the neurobehavioral mechanisms underlying the efficacy of the new drugs, should of course, be put to use in the development of new antidepressants and in redesigning the clinical trial of the future to better evaluate these new agents. It is as if the results of the hundreds of clinical trials conducted during this period, although successful in rare cases of identifying new efficacious drugs, have provided extremely limited information about the actions of these many drugs. We know only whether they were effective or ineffective in resolving the targeted depressive disorders. Despite the great expense and great effort expended, no other reliable information has resulted that would expand knowledge and information on the impact of these chemical agents on the clinical aspects of psychopathology. No network of important information on their profiles of behavioral actions exists. Nor have the correlations of those actions with the effects on neurochemistry been assembled, information of obvious value in the design of new treatment drugs. Such information is critical for the clinician in potentially finding applications of these drugs for the treatment of other mental disorders, or to provide information toward improving their management of treatments. Critics would certainly view the conventional clinical trial as not only outdated from the standpoint of recent research advances, but exceedingly wasteful in its mode of research operations.

In the next chapter, I present an example of the proposed new model which would in fact, take advantage of this new information based on decades of research and make more effective use of the high expense in funds, time and effort that go into creating and conducting a clinical trial.

Chapter 3
Reconceptualizing Depression, and the Current Scene on Dimensionality and the RDoC

The foundation for developing a new approach to clinical trials lies in a rethinking and possibly, a new conceptualization of the disorder itself, in light of the advances in neurobiology during the past five decades. So that different from earlier, we now when examining its phenomenology must take into account its associations with the dysfunctioning of central neurotransmitter systems, and ask how these dysfunctions relate to the mood and behavioral disturbance manifest in its clinical presentation. In our own research efforts (Maas et al. 1980) that sought to uncover these associations, we learned that increasing the availability of serotonin and norepinephrine in neural functioning led to specific changes in anxiety, motor retardation and depressed mood in classical clinical cases (Katz et al. 1994). To learn more about the underlying mechanisms and how the drugs resolved those disorders, it was clear that we would have to clarify these associations between the elements of the neurochemical systems and its behavioral components.

We were convinced that the drugs were not "diagnosis-specific" in their actions, but "component-specific". The immediate tasks, therefore, were to identify the behavioral elements of the disorder so as to determine the nature of the associations between the neural and behavioral systems. To this end we reexamined the clinical nature, i.e., the behavioral and symptomatic characteristics of a large and diverse sample of soundly diagnosed major depressive disorders (MDDs) (130 patients from six hospitals) through use of a range of behavioral methods, including observational ratings by clinicians and nurses, self ratings by patients and a battery of psychomotor performance tests. The instruments were designed to cover all domains of symptomatology and expression identified earlier in such comprehensive and sound analyses of the phenomenology in studies by Grinker et al. (1960) and Kendell (1968). Through use of the battery we were able to measure all relevant facets on the 150 depressed and manic patients and 80 normal controls and to submit the data to a principal components analysis (Hotelling 1933). That analysis both described eleven behavior, mood, cognitive and somatic

© The Author(s) 2016
M.M. Katz, *Clinical Trials of Antidepressants*, SpringerBriefs in Psychology,
DOI 10.1007/978-3-319-26464-6_3

components and generated the principal factors or dimensions that underlie their associations (Katz et al. 1984). That analysis did in other words, uncover the behavioral and emotional structure. We identified three independent dimensions that were capable of explaining 75 % of the variance among the components. The three were: depressed mood-motor retardation, anxiety-agitation-somatization, and hostility-interpersonal sensitivity. Of the components not included in the dimensions were "distressed expression" based on the subject's physical expression and "cognitive impairment" that was associated equally with the first two dimensions.

Thus, we had quantified measures, based on analyses of data from validated methods that provided a profile of dimensions and elemental components of the major depressive disorder (unipolar and bipolar). We would then examine the nature of the disorder through these elements and determine how they were associated with the neurochemical elements, and possibly, uncover the neurobehavioral mechanisms underlying the disorder and the efficacy of the antidepressant drugs.

Here is what we found on our way to "rethinking" the nature of the depressive disorder.

The profile of the typical patient diagnosed with an acute "major depressive disorder" will show high levels both on the anxiety-agitation and depressed mood—retardation dimensions with significantly, but not as high levels on the hostility dimension and cognitive impairment (see Fig. 3.1). It is common knowledge, from long experience with this clinical condition, that a high level of anxiety

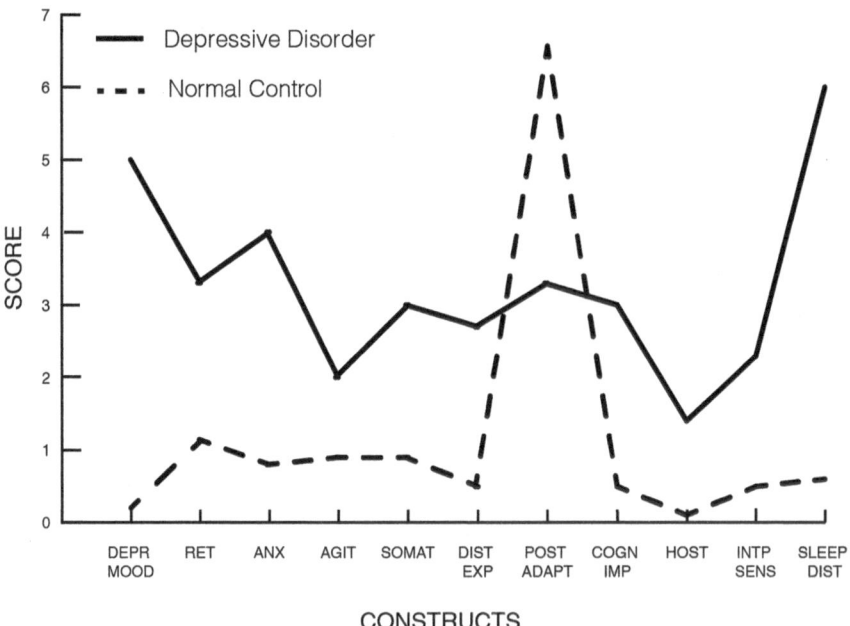

Fig. 3.1 Depressive disorders and normal controls: baseline patterns of behavioral and affect constructs. Reproduced with permission of publisher from Katz et al. (1984). © Psychological Reports 1984

accompanies the depressed mood and retardation, and that feelings of anger existent in most patients, are less visible at first, but undoubtedly present. Although the dimensions of depressed mood and anxiety are significantly correlated, our work identifies these dimensions as generated from potentially, independent sources. An analysis of their relationships with central neurotransmitter dysfunctions informs that they are different, i.e., the level of anxiety associated more directly with the serotonin system, the depressed mood-retardation, with the noradrenergic system. The patterns of relationships are not so clear as to be described currently in more precise terms, but the fact that theses patterns are different, is now supported by strong laboratory evidence (Morilak and Frazer 2004).

"Opposed Neurobehavioral States"

We proceeded in our interpretation of these neural and behavioral relationships to hypothesize that the dimensions, depressed mood-retardation, anxiety-agitation, and hostility represented three different, partially overlapping neurobehavioral states, each of which is dysfunctional in the depressive disorder. From that standpoint, and as presented with more detailed background in my recent book (Katz 2013), the dimensions, depressed—mood-retardation and anxiety-agitation represent "opposed" neuroemotional states of the central nervous system (CNS). The former dimension reflects a sedated, energyless state, the latter, a state of "arousal", one more motorically active. The patient, in part, the "victim" of this profile, aside from its other components, would experience this apparent clash of emotional states and thus, be subjected to the further turmoil this conflict introduces. I designated this new hypothesis (theory) relative to its clinical nature as one of "conflicting neurobehavioral states" that further exacerbates the inner turmoil that patients suffer with in this experience of the disorder.

How then does this "redefining" of the acute depressive disorder affect how we evaluate new potential antidepressant treatments? One need not accept the above theoretical interpretation in its entirety. This new vantage point, however, underlines the importance of identifying the basic dimensions and components, and then directs the search for drugs that target these dimensions, i.e., drugs that specifically target anxiety, motor activity, depressed mood or hostility, as against attempting to target the disorder as a "whole".

To evaluate the profile of the actions of the trial drug on behavioral, mood, somatic and cognitive components, it is, therefore, necessary to supplement the Ham-D with the prescribed additional behavioral methodology. It can be seen now that the two major changes necessary in any remodeling of the clinical trial, based on research advances during the past several decades, are (1) to target dimensions, not diagnosis and (2) to provide a profile of the trial drug actions on behavior, mood and cognition, a profile that can be placed alongside that of the drug's actions on central neurotransmitter systems.

On Replacing Diagnosis with Dimensions: The Current Scene and the RDoC

It is of interest, that the dimensionality concept has in recent years begun to gain traction both as regards the basis for diagnosis of the mental disorders, as reflected in its limited role in the new DSM-5 (2014) and as the foundation for the ongoing development of a wholly new, more comprehensive approach to classification of the disorders, the Research Domain Criteria (RDoC) (Cuthbert and Insel 2010). Regarding the DSM-5, it appears that dimensionality is only applied to the severity of core symptoms in schizophrenia as a replacement in the system for the now eliminated traditional subtypes of the disorder. The RDoC will, however, over the next several years, provide a classification of disorders based on the dimensions that encompass all validated neuroscientific and psychopathologic elements, so far uncovered in these sciences. We look forward to this development which will undoubtedly put diagnosis on a much firmer and more informative base and specifically, serve purposes of research in the field, currently not well served by the established diagnostic system.

The drawbacks of these developments on the current scene are that dimensionality will as noted, play a very small role in the DSM-5 and as important an advance as the RDoC will be, in 2015 it remains a work in progress.The results from research in developing the system are not likely to be available to apply for several years. In the interim, it is, recommended that the current multivantaged (MV) system that has already demonstrated utility in quantifying the major facets and sensitivity in detecting specific clinical actions of the new drugs, be applied in current investigations in clinical psychopharmacology.

It will also be sometime before the Food and drug Administration (FDA) that takes its lead from psychiatry and the drug industry can replace, or modify the diagnostic approach with dimensions. Their requirement that there be two positive trials conducted with the randomized, control study model, still rightfully meets, as it should, the importance of demonstrating non-bias in response to the question of efficacy in the clinical trial.

Chapter 4
Aims and Basic Requirements of Clinical Trials: Conventional and Component-Specific Models

In March 2004 the periodical, the Economist, in its quarterly analysis of technology, reviewed advances in psychopharmacology, citing that despite the doubling of research funds since 1991 and the abundance of new biotechnical tools, most drug discovery and development efforts still fail. New drugs emerging each year (since 1991) have fallen by half. They raised the question, Why? The main reason cited was: "because of a lack of understanding of how they work." A Task Force of the Collegium Internationale of Neuropsychopharmacology (CINP) convened at about that time also, for more scientifically based reasons, came to the same conclusion (Sartorius et al. 2007).

Why was this the case? In contrast to the early trials of the tricyclic andtidepressants in the 1960s, there was now a declining capacity to show a new, putative AD to be superior in efficacy to a placebo. Certain of the methodologic issues associated with changes in studies during this period can be cited as causes for these failures: (1) There was a movement of type of settings for clinical trial studies, from hospital to outpatient settings. (2) The target populations now studied were less severely ill than the earlier patients who were for the most part, hospitalized. (3) The sole methods of evaluating the new drugs lack sensitivity to most of the drug-induced changes in the less severely ill, many changes of which occur in components of the disorder. (4) Placebo treatment is more effective in the less than most severely ill, thus, creating a new problem, requiring greater sensitivity and statistical power in the evaluation process.

These problems require investigators to adapt to these changes in the target population and to consider the need for greater sensitivity in the evaluation process and to redesign the trial, generally. In order to determine how best to go about the restructuring of a trial, I describe two models for evaluation, the established diagnosis-specific and the component-specific. The latter is adapted specifically, to deal with the current set of new problems in this area (Table 4.1).

© The Author(s) 2016
M.M. Katz, *Clinical Trials of Antidepressants*, SpringerBriefs in Psychology,
DOI 10.1007/978-3-319-26464-6_4

Table 4.1 Models for design of antidepressant trials: disorder-specific versus component-specific

---

Disorder-specific: Based on theory that depression is a unitary disorder caused by a dysfunction in central nervous system chemistry. The "antidepressant" drug is presumed to target the specific pathophysiology underlying the disorder. A test of the drug's efficacy then requires measuring its capacity to reduce the severity of the "whole" syndrome and to possibly, eliminate the disorder. The most effective methods for measuring changes in the severity and overall treatment outcome used are the Hamilton Depression Rating Scale (1960) and the MADRS (Montgomery and Asberg 1979)

Component-specific: Research indicates that the central neurotransmitter systems presumed to be associated with the pathology of depression are the serotonergic and noradrenergic systems. Basic research links these systems with the regulation of different behaviors and moods, serotonin with impulsive aggression and anxiety, norepinephrine with" arousal" and motor activity. Antidepressants have been found to be equally effective for anxiety, phobic and obsessive-compulsive disorders. Thus, their therapeutic effects in depression are more likely based on the changes they effect in the components of anxiety, hostility and motor functioning, not necessarily in the "core" pathology of depression. The most effective methods for measuring drug action are methods for measuring the principal behavioral, mood and cognitive components of the disorder (Katz and Maas 1994)

I note regarding the primary aim of the AD clinical trial that it has not changed. It is to evaluate the efficacy of a new drug in the treatment of the major depressive disorder. In view of the multiyear, multidisciplinary effort involved in the development of the new treatment agent and the vast expense associated with clinical evaluation, it is important toward advancing the science of psychopharmacology and to provide a profile of the nature and sequence of clinical actions of a putative antidepressant, to incorporate a set of secondary aims for the trial. The secondary aims are:

1. Identifying the initial actions of the drug.
2. Determining the onset and timing of drug-induced clinical actions.
3. Characterizing its behavioral, mood, cognitive and somatic actions.
4. Predicting clinical response at outcome.
5. Identifying potential applications of the new drug to the treatment of other mental disorders.

The component-specific model is based on the premise that the major depressive disorder is not unitary, but multi-faceted, comprised of major behavioral and affective components that interact to create the disordered state.

Empirical studies of the phenomena of the disorder, carried out by Grinker et al. (1961), Kendell (1968), Maas et al. (1980), Katz et al. (1984, 2004) identified the major behavioral, mood, cognitive and somatic components.

When considering how well these models, the established diagnosis-specific and the componential model achieve the primary aim, we note that both are highly effective. However, when the patient sample is less severely ill, in the range of marked to mild depression, when symptomatology is less manifest, evaluation requires both more intensive observation and more extensive inquiry. In this case, the diagnosis-specific model that relies exclusively on observational judgment for measurement of change in overall severity of the disorder, is not as effective or as sensitive in detecting specific clinical actions as the component-specific model.

When comparing the models in regard to achieving the secondary aims, it is clear that the measurement of specific drug clinical actions must be intensified. The diagnosis-specific model is not designed to provide refined measurement of the specific clinical actions of ADs on mood, behavior and cognitive components. Measurement of changes in symptoms, e.g., are confined to Ham-D or MADRS items, highly insensitive and unreliable measures of the facets of the disorder.

Herein lies the problem of why despite major advances in measuring drug-induced changes in neurochemistry, the measurement of changes in clinical phenomena has lagged badly behind. The failure to use the component-specific model has deprived the field of accurate knowledge on the timing and onset of clinical actions, the capacity to predict clinical response at outcome, and describing differences in action between pharmacologically different drugs (Katz et al. 2004).

That is why we were not able to provide the answers to the queries raised by the Economist in 2004 as to how the drugs initiate and sustain a specific set of clinical actions, what the mechanisms are that underlie their efficacy.

Toward successfully achieving the secondary aims, it is clear that the componential is superior to the diagnostic-specific model. In the next chapter 1 describe the multivantage approach (MV) (Katz et al. 2004), i.e., the set of behavioral methods designed to measure changes in overall severity, the primary aim of the clinical trial. It will in addition, measure changes in the behavioral components, actions essential to achieving the secondary aims.

Chapter 5
Methods for Measuring the Components and the Profile of Drug Actions: The Multivantaged Approach

The general approach is to apply methods that in addition to measuring overall severity of the targeted disorder, will also provide sound measures of each of the major components. To accomplish that, several types of measurement must be applied: observational ratings (by clinicians, nurses and trained observers); direct self-report by the patient, and psychomotor performance tests. One validated method set of this type is drawn from the NIMH Collaborative Study of the Psychobiology of Depression (Maas et al. 1980). Overall severity, the depressed mood-motor retardation, arousal and hostility dimensions and measures of the associated components are drawn from the data on 130 diagnosed depressed patients and smaller control samples of manic patients and healthy controls.

It is important drawing from earlier discussions of the background of this approach to identify the assumptions that underlie the original and established clinical trials of putative antidepressants. Against that background we can determine what scientific evidence assembled over the last several decades has to tell us about the accuracy of these early assumptions. I do that by assembling in Table 5.1 a list of the assumptions in the left hand column and the evidence in the right hand column.

It can be seen from the comparison in Table 5.1 that the assumptions that formed the basis for designing the clinical trials of new antidepressants in the 1950s and early 1960s, have for the most part, been proven invalid. Recently collected evidence presents a very different picture of the structure of the basic disorder that is targeted for treatment and the nature and sequence of drug actions that induce clinical changes.

The ADs are not diagnostic-specific. They apparently, through effects on the various central neurotransmitter systems induce changes in the behavioral components, e.g., on anxiety, hostility, depressed mood and motor activity. How these behavioral components are affected is a function of the pattern of actions on neurotransmitter systems, which in themselves, have different patterns of associations

© The Author(s) 2016
M.M. Katz, *Clinical Trials of Antidepressants*, SpringerBriefs in Psychology,
DOI 10.1007/978-3-319-26464-6_5

Table 5.1 Assumptions that guided early trials versus evidence-based findings

Assumptions	Evidence-based findings
1. ADs are specific for treatment of depressive disorders	1. ADs are specific for reducing anxiety, hostility, motor retardation, depressed mood
2. AD-induced clinical actions lag several weeks behind almost immediate effects on neurotransmitter systems. Quitkin et al. (1984)	2. ADs initiate improvement in anxiety and hostility within the 1st 2 weeks; full response in 6–8
3. Pharmacologically different ADs initially affect the same symptoms in responsive patients. Nelson et al. (1999)	3. Pharmacologically different ADs induce different treatment-sequences of behavioral and mood changes prior to resulting in full response
4. Depression is a unitary disorder with depressed mood and retardation reflected in its core dimensions	4. Depression is multifaceted in composition, comprised mainly of the interaction of 3 dimensions anxiety-agitation, depressed mood-motor retardation, and hostility

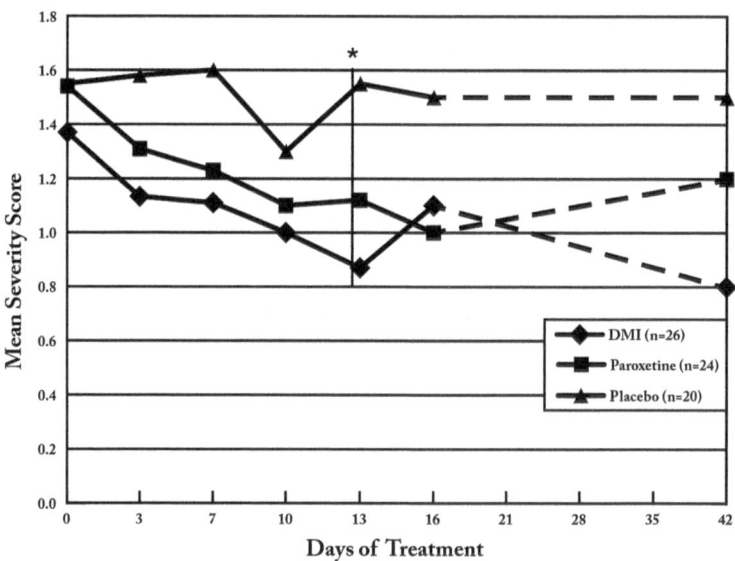

Fig. 5.1 *Early drug actions*: comparing treatments across time periods on hostility. DMI and paroxetine reduce hostility at a significantly faster rate during the first 2 weeks than placebo (slopes test $p < 0.05$). At day 13 of treatment DMI improved hostility significantly more than placebo *$p < 0.05$, ANCOVA). Reproduced with permission of publisher from Katz et al. (2004). © Neuropsychopharmacology 2004

with the array of behavioral components. We learn that with more refined measurement, the drug induced actions on clinical aspects occur earlier than originally thought in the treatment process and that effective ADs having different neurochemical characteristics induce different patterns of symptomatic and behavioral changes in treatment-responsive patients.

For example, the onset of clinical actions of the TCAs, the SSRIs, and selective noradrenergic drugs on major components of the disorder in treatment-responsive patients is 7–14 days, not several weeks as commonly reported in earlier

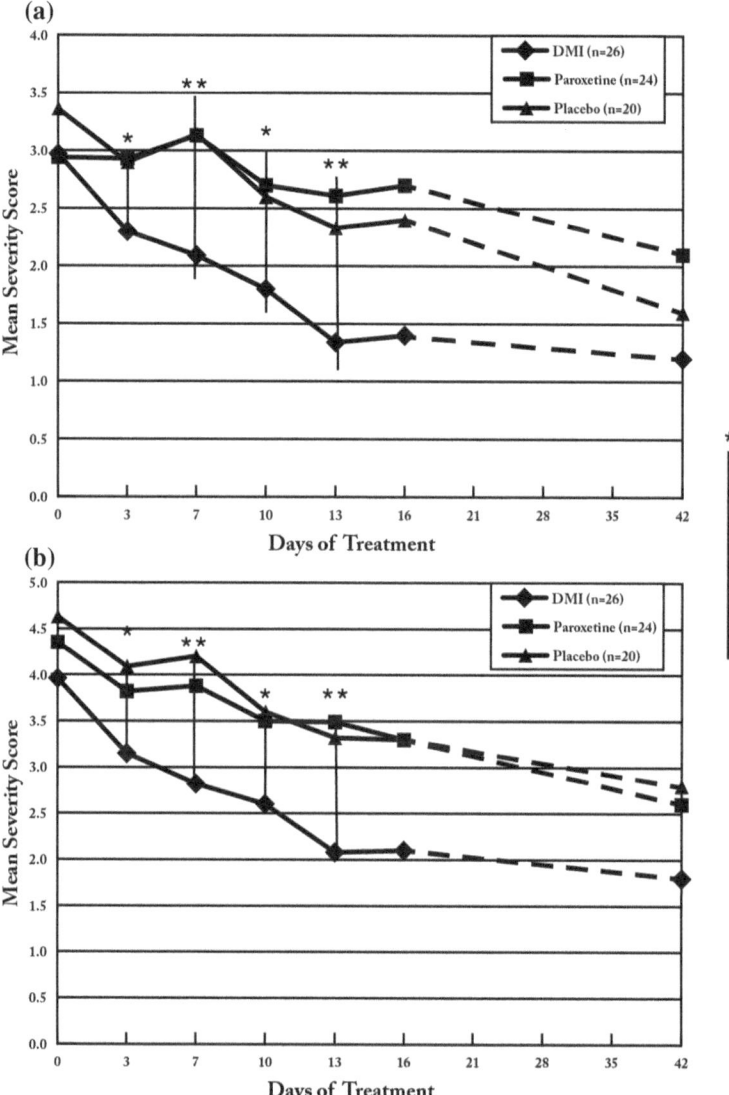

Fig. 5.2 *Early drug actions*: comparing DMI, paroxetine, and placebo across time periods. **a** *Motor retardation*: at days 7 and 13 of treatment DMI improved motor retardation significantly more than that caused by either paroxetine or placebo (**$p < 0.01$, ANCOVA) and at day 10, the same effect was observed (*$p < 0.05$, ANCOVA). **b** *Severity dimension*: DM-MR at days 7 and 13 of treatment DMI improved the severity dimension significantly more than that due to either paroxetine or placebo (**$p < 0.01$, ANCOVA) and at day 10, the improvement caused by DMI was significantly greater than that caused by paroxetine (*$p < 0.05$, ANCOVA). Although behavioral assessments were conducted at days 21, 28, and 35 of treatment these time points were not essential for the hypothesis being tested. Consequently, values obtained at these time points are omitted from Figs. 3.1a, b and 5.1 for the clarity of data presentation. Reproduced with permission of publisher from Katz et al. (2004). © Neuropychopharmacology 2004

textbooks. The more recent findings of earlier clinical actions have been confirmed in independent studies (Katz et al. 2004) and in several metaanalyses of clinical trial results (Stassen et al. 1996; Szegedi et al. 2009).

To illustrate these changes, see Figs. 5.1 and 5.2 (Onset and Early behavioral actions of ADs):

They compare a representative TCA (desipramine) actions with those of an SSRI (paroxetine).

Note also the result of such studies as Stassen et al. (1997) that shows early improvement (EI) to occur in 70 % of AD treatment responders.

And Posternak and Zimmerman (2005) that showed 60 % of improvement that occurred on medication as occurring during the first week of treatment.

In Appendix II the components and dimensions based on the empirical studies described earlier are listed. The methods selected to measure them and on which they are based are in Appendix IV. The list of methods and the times required for the administration of each are displayed.

Details on each of these methods, i.e., the psychometric studies that established their reliability and validity in measuring components has been presented in prior publications, the 1984 monograph (Katz et al.) and in the paper which described the brief battery in Katz et al. (2004).

To ease understanding, the methods designed for observational ratings of inter-view behavior, self-reports and psychomotor performance are briefly described as is their application in the measurement of specific components in the MV battery. It can be seen that the components cover moods and feelings, depression, anxi-ety, and hostility or feeling of anger, motor activity, retarded or agitated, cogni-tive impairment, somatic complaints, sleep disturbance and distressed physical expression.

The moods are assessed from the vantages of the clinicians (Ham-D, SADS-C (Endicott et al. 1978), NIMH Mood (Raskin et al. 1969) and the patient (NIMH Mood scale, SCL-90, Derogatis et al. 1979), motor activity (clinical observation through SADS-C, Ham-D), patient performance (psychomotor tests, physical expression (VIBES) (Katz et al. 2006), cognitive impairment (Dr. and patient rat-ings on SADS-C and NIMH Mood) and somatic complaints (SADS-C, SCL-90). Examples of the administration of the Multivantage and Video models in actual patient cases are in Appendix I. It includes records of the before treatment, during and after interviews and resultant construct scores for four sample patients. They were selected to illustrate three patients who changed markedly, but differently, during treatment and a fourth, who showed little to no response to the experimen-tal drug.

From application of these procedures during the course of treatment, we learn that different drugs result in different sequences of behavioral change. These results are best illustrated by describing an example of a "component-specific" trial, one which compares two classes of drug (e.g., SSRI and SNRI) and placebo, followed by a comparison of its results with those obtained if the clinical trial con-ducted was based on the established diagnosis-specific model in which the sole method of clinical evaluation was the Ham-D.

Chapter 6
Achieving the "Ideal" Clinical Trial: An Example of Applying the Merged Componential and Established Models

The current ideal clinical trial would be one that incorporates the MV model and the conventional, currently established, Hamilton-D model.

In the example to be used in this chapter, the Video model, although it can stand on its own as a trial method, can be added to the design, as described. Thus, a trial that integrated all 3 models, would in my judgment, represent the ideal for the field.

Why? To answer, I have to return to an earlier theme and restate the basis for this thinking.

The current established procedure for the conduct of the clinical trial is a vastly expensive use of resources that is designed solely to determine the overall efficacy and the potential marketability of that new treatment. This occurs in the context of an active scientific field devoted to investigating the underlying neurobehavioral mechanisms of drug actions and developing novel treatments for the targeted disorders. That context requires new information on the nature of the neurobehavioral condition itself, and of the mechanisms underlying the efficacy of already established treatments. It requires this information in order to develop new, more effective, more rapidly acting drugs to treat the disorders.

To conduct a conventional trial costs at minimum, hundreds of thousands of dollars, and only indicates whether a drug is efficacious for a targeted disorder. Granted the importance of this goal for clinical practice, it means that added opportunities to uncover new information about basic mechanisms, how and why such drugs do or do not work, are completely unattended. In other words, achieving the secondary or scientific aims of such a study, i.e., analysis of the interaction of the elements of treatment and of the disorder, are completely lost.

If there should be any signs of unexpected activity of the new drug, e.g., on any of the other critical aspects of the disorder, such as the level of anxiety or of repressed anger in the context of the depressive disorder, a new study, probably equally expensive, would have then to be developed and new funding sought to conduct it.

© The Author(s) 2016

M.M. Katz, *Clinical Trials of Antidepressants*, SpringerBriefs in Psychology, DOI 10.1007/978-3-319-26464-6_6

By adding little additional methodology to the established trial, i.e., adopting the MV model, the secondary, scientific aims of the study would be achieved. Both the primary and secondary goals can then, be accomplished within the framework of the clinical trial. In this and in the next chapter, I provide a concrete example of this approach and the results it can produce.

The "essence" of what is proposed here is that we convert the "clinical trial" into a "scientific, clinical study" aimed at achieving both the practical, primary aim of determining whether the new drug is efficacious for the targeted disorder, and the secondary, scientific aims of describing the nature and timing of the full range of clinical actions the drug has on the major aspects of the depressive disorder.

It will be noted in the example to follow that although one may continue to think in the traditional manner that the depressive disorder is "holistic", unitary in nature with a core depressive syndrome, that it is necessary in the context of this study to adopt a dimensional concept of the disorder. Here for the purpose of the research, the disorder is conceived of as comprised of several major components, that as the author has demonstrated in prior studies, based on a structure that consists of the interaction of several major components of affect, cognition, motor activity and somatic involvement.

Applying the Models

Here I describe a study conducted in the late 1990s, then later published (Katz et al. 2004). It was designed to determine the time of onset of improvement induced by representatives of two different classes of drugs, a tricyclic noradrenergic targeted drug, desipramine (DMI), and an SSRI, paroxetine, and their respective sequences and profiles of clinical actions. The study included a placebo treated control. The study was not specifically designed as a clinical trial, since both drugs had already been established in earlier studies, as efficacious antidepressants. The study would, however, have all the requirements necessary to be interpreted as a trial and could serve, although the patient sample is modest in size, as a model of the component-specific trial and provide results that could be compared with the results from conducting a study in accord with the conventional model. Further, since the MV method also incorporates the Ham-D, the results of the componential study could then be compared directly with the established Ham-D model.

Here are the specifics of that study: **Design**: The structure entailed random assignment of patients diagnosed "major depressive disorder" to parallel groups, "double blind" assignment of incoming patients to DMI, paroxetine or placebo for a treatment period of six weeks. The patients were both hospitalized and outpatient, drawn from VA facilities. All were interviewed initially with the standardized procedure, the DSM III SCID (Spitzer and Williams 1983) and subsequently, diagnosed as major depressive disorders (MDD), unipolar type, and all required to have a Ham-D baseline score of ≥ 18 (21 item version).

Patient Sample: A total of 82 patients were initially enrolled and randomly assigned to treatment. Of these 12 patients dropped out for various reasons prior to receiving the three minimum weeks of treatment. A total of 70 patients completed the protocol (58 male, 12 female, average age of 46, range 20–69). Most patients were moderately ill (56 %), 38 %, severely ill. as rated on the Clinical Global Improvement Scale (CGI), (Guy 1976). The average Ham-D at baseline was $23.5 + 4.5$ (Mean + SD), with scores essentially the same at the two research sites, San Antonio and Dallas.

Baseline and Treatment Period: An initial 7 day drug "washout" period was required. Prior to starting treatment patients had to show ≥ 18 score on the Ham-D. Patients assigned to DMI were started at 50 mg and raised as necessary to a maximum of 350 mg/day in order to reach a blood level of >125 ng/ml by 7 days. Steady state concentrations of DMI were reached by 13 days for 80 % of the 29 patients assigned to DMI. Of these patients three dropped out due to side effects. Dosage for paroxetine ranged from 20 to 60 mg/day, adjusted to achieve a minimum steady state serum concentration of at least 10 ng/ml, reached by day 6 for 94 % of patients.

A total of 25 patients were assigned to placebo; five did not complete the minimum of 3 weeks in protocol. The final total of all patients following exclusion of all who did not complete 3 weeks of treatment was 70.

Measurement of Behavioral Components and Severity of Depressed State

The list of methods are in Appendix III; they were designed to measure specific behavioral components and overall severity of the disorder in order to address questions of onset and comparability of the behavioral changes induced by the pharmacologically different drugs, DMI and paroxetine.

It is of interest that since the time of that study more clinical trials have started to add behavioral methodology, particularly, regarding cognitive and motor functioning, e.g., see review of studies by Rosenthal et al. (2015). These studies used a wide range of cognitive methods but despite the number and range of techniques applied, the results that showed drug actions in this area of psychological functioning, were minimal. The MV method used in the Texas study (2004) covers an even broader range of functioning including measures of cognition and motor activity, but administers techniques that had in past studies, demonstrated significant sensitivity to drug effects.

To achieve the **primary and secondary aims of the clinical trial**:

1. the drugs were compared on efficacy for MDD at 6 weeks.
2. the time of onset and the nature and sequence of drug-induced changes were determined by identifying initial actions of the drug.

3. It was determined whether the pharmacologically different drugs differed in the pattern of clinical actions, in the change in the profile of actions they induced in depressed patients, i.e., how they brought about efficacy in treating MDD.
4. Whether specific early changes, i.e., within the first 2 weeks, were predictive of clinical response at outcome.

To measure overall efficacy of the experimental drugs, they were compared with placebo at 6 weeks on the established method for measuring change in the severity of the overall disorder, specifically ≥50 % decrease in the Ham-D scale or direct analysis of covariance using baseline values as controls. The results as reported in Katz et al. 2004 are (a) DMI showed a 62 % response rate at 6 weeks indicating significantly more efficacy than placebo and paroxetine which showed 46 and 45 % response rates, respectively. Paroxetine was, therefore, not found to be significantly more effective than placebo. (b) By the end of week 1, DMI decreased the dimension depressed mood-motor retardation and the specific components significantly more than placebo and paroxetine and by week 2, added to that a significantly greater reduction in hostility, when compared with the other treatments. (c) At 10 days, paroxetine reduced anxiety significantly more than did placebo. At two weeks, a slopes analysis (Laird and Ware 1982) showed both DMI and paroxetine to reduce hostility significantly more rapidly than did placebo.

Onset for clinical change for DMI was therefore, as early as one week, specifically on the dimension of depressed mood-retardation; paroxetine, on anxiety at 10 days, and with DMI on hostility by two weeks.

Although paroxetine overall was not significantly more efficacious than placebo (primarily due to the majority of males in the sample, as analysed in the 2004 paper), in those patients who responded to the drug, the behavioral changes differed in nature and sequence from those described in responders to DMI. For example, the initial changes in paroxetine were in reductions in anxiety and hostility, for DMI in depressed mood-retardation.

The range of these effects in individual cases are graphically illustrated in the sample patients drawn from the Collaborative and Texas studies and described in Appendix I. The descriptions will be helpful in interpreting the overall results. Were these early drug-induced changes (at 2 weeks). e.g., predictive of full response to the drug at six week outcome? A logistic regression analysis showed they were with DMI. When using only the DM-MR dimension, the combined sensitivity and specificity was at 0.90 and 0.88, respectively; for paroxetine, based on combined components at 2 weeks, the sensitivity and specificity were 0.85 and 0.91, respectively.

The conclusions here are that the primary and all secondary aims of the clinical trial were achieved, resulting in evidence-based conclusions on efficacy, onset, nature and time of clinical actions, in addition to the potential capacity to predict clinical response at outcome at 6 weeks, following two weeks of treatment.

One can refer to further detail of the study and discussion of the results, particularly as they relate to the targeted actions of the selective ADs on the central neurotransmitter systems and their specific associations with the behavioral, mood and somatic components of the clinical profile in the Katz et al. 2004 paper. The intention here was to view the study as an example of how a sample clinical trial, complete with the requirements of the proposed "component-specific" model, would be designed, conducted and the resulting data analysed.

In the next chapter, I compare results of the new model with the established Ham-D model and attempt to characterize the significant advantages that the component-specific offers.

Chapter 7
Comparing the Component-Specific Model Directly with the Established Diagnosis-Specific Trial

Earlier I outlined the primary and secondary aims of the model clinical trial of new putative antidepressants. In this chapter, the componential and the established diagnosis-specific trials are compared on how well each of the aims are achieved.

Regarding the critical **primary aim**, i.e., determining whether the experimental drug is efficacious, using the 2004 study as an example, we find that either system, the diagnosis-specific that utilizes the Ham-D as the sole method for clinical evaluation, or the component-specific, can successfully and validly answer the question.

In the 2004 study, the traditional efficacy measure of a ≥ 50 % decrease in the Ham-D total score, resulted in a significantly greater improvement for DMI versus placebo, when that index was applied in either of the clinical trial models. This was not the case for the paroxetine versus placebo comparison. Reasons as to why paroxetine already established in earlier trials as an effective antidepressant, was not shown to be in this study are cited in the Katz et al. 2004 paper. It was suggested, e.g., that the lower response rate for paroxetine in this study as compared with others, was due to most of the depressed patients in the 2004 study being male. Earlier studies (Korstein et al. 2000; Joyce et al. 2003) showed men to respond less well to SSRIs than to TCAs. In those studies the response rates of males to SSRIs was about 40–45 %, similar to the response rate in this study of 46 %. By contrast, response rate to DMI in the 2004 study was 62 %. Since both models utilized the Ham-D, both were equally capable of achieving the primary aim, i.e., determining the efficacy or non-efficacy of the trial drugs.

Secondary Aims

Profiles of clinical actions, onset and timing of actions.

© The Author(s) 2016
M.M. Katz, *Clinical Trials of Antidepressants*, SpringerBriefs in Psychology,
DOI 10.1007/978-3-319-26464-6_7

Table 7.1 Time of onset[a]
of improvement in treatment
responders (survival analysis)

	Day of onset		
	DMI	Paroxetine	Placebo
State constructs			
Depressed mood	3	13	16
Anxiety	7	10	16
Motor retardation	7	13	21
Distressed expression	13	13	42
Severity			
Hamilton Scale	7	10	10
DM-MR dimension	3	13	21

Reproduced with permission of publisher from Katz et al. (2004). © Neuropsychopharmacology 2004

[a]*Onset* Time point (days of treatment) at which ≥ 50 % of patients show ≥ 20 % of improvement that is sustained through 6 weeks of treatment

Regarding these aims, it is clear that the disorder-specific trial conducted in the conventional manner might, if assessments are conducted on a weekly basis, provide information on onset of overall clinical action. It would not, confined as it is to the total Ham-D score, although a valid index of changes in the severity of the overall disorder, be able to provide reliable measures on components or provide a profile of the specific drug-induced actions and the sequence of these actions, the other secondary aims of the clinical trial.

On onset, we learn that the Ham-D significantly detected change, i.e., ≥ 20 % decrease in total score, at one week of treatment. The "component-specific" analysis, which includes finding the Ham-D onset at 7 days, also shows for DMI, specific clinical changes beginning at 3 days on the depressed mood component and the depressed mood-retardation dimension, and changes on the anxiety and motor retardation components at 7 days (see Table 7.1).

The Ham-D 20 % reduction occurred at 10 days for paroxetine, apparently due primarily, to the decrease in the anxiety component, also shown in the "component-specific" analysis to be significantly reduced at that onset point in treatment-responsive patients. The Ham-D also detected onset in placebo responders at 10 days, but no specific componential actions until 16 days (then acted on depressed mood and anxiety).

Conclusions here as to how well the models compare inform that although the Ham-D can contribute to estimating time of onset of clinical action, as within the first week of treatment, it is significantly less sensitive than the component-specific, which shows certain components demonstrating significant changes as early as 3 days.

These changes are illustrated in Table 7.1.

On others of the secondary aims, the established "disorder-specific" has little to show due to the absence of any methods for measuring changes in the major components or dimensions of the disorder.

Therefore, such aims as identifying drug-induced, specific clinical actions, the timing and sequence of such drug-induced actions that may identify drug actions that are potentially applicable to the treatment of other mental disorders, are beyond what can be achieved through application of the established disorder-specific clinical trial.

Here through applying the "component-specific", we learn the following regarding the secondary aims:

The initial clinical actions induced by DMI are on depressed mood-retardation, as early as 3 days, followed quickly by reductions in anxiety and hostility.

Thus, through application of the component-specific trial, we achieve a profile of initial drug-induced clinical actions along with sequence of these actions followed over the course of treatment. We note again how important it is to achieve these secondary aims of the clinical trials. They contribute at the basic level, to more refined understanding of the relationships between actions of the drugs on selected neurotransmitter systems and their effects on behavior, e.g., the effects of DMI as a noradrenergic selective drug, is to increase the availability of norepinephrine and the demonstration of norepinephrine's association with "arousal", alertness, engagement of the organism in its external environment, behavior which clinicians, as early as Kielholz and Poldinger (1968) recognized to be an effect of the TCAs. Here in the 2004 study the association is demonstrated as we note between the initial effects of DMI on the reduction of "motor retardation" and "depressed mood" (Table 7.2).

Table 7.2 Results from applying componential approach compared with established diagnosis-specific trial

1.	**On specificity and clinical actions**
	The initial actions of the TCAs and SSRIs are on the components of anxiety and hostility, for the selective noradrenergic drug (DMI), on motor activity and anxiety
	See Figs. 5.1 and 5.2 comparing SSRI and SNRI and with placebo on motor retardation and hostility
2.	**Onset and timing of drug actions**
	The onset of the clinical actions of TCAs, SSRIs, and selective noradrenergic drugs on major components of the disorder in treatment—responsive patients is 7–14 days, not several weeks as commonly reported in most textbooks. The most recent findings of earlier action have been confirmed in clinical studies and in meta-analyses of clinical trials results. Results from the latter studies that utilized the Ham-D were reanalyzed using survival analysis to estimate time of onset of initial improvement
3.	**Prediction of clinical response**
	Absence of behavioral changes during first two to three weeks of treatment with an AD is highly associated with non-clinical response at outcome
	Taylor et al. (2006) "one-third of the total effect of SSRIs after 6 weeks of treatment is seen in the first week"
	Stassen et al. (1997) "among responders the onset of improvement occurs in more than 70 % of cases within the first three weeks", on average, no more than 10 % of patients who do not show any improvement within the first three weeks will become treatment responders"
	Katz et al. (2004) "drug-specific types of behavioral response in the first one or two weeks of treatment with DMI or paroxetine are highly predictive of six week outcome"

Posternak and Zimmerman (2005) "60.2 and 61.6 % of the improvement that occurred on active medication and placebo, respectively, took place during the first two weeks of treatment

At the clinical level we note the effects of the SSRIs on anxiety, again an effect that might have been predicted based on the research that demonstrated the significant association between serotonin and anxiety (Dunbar and Fuell 1992), later helping to open the possibility of applying the SSRIs to the treatment of anxiety disorders. It was then demonstrated to be more effective than the benzodiazepines for treating the generalized anxiety type of the disorder (Kahn et al. 1989).

Further, ability to determine time of onset and the therapeutic actions of new drugs, i.e., within 2 weeks of treatment, information that the component-specific trial provides, makes it possible to predict outcome within that early time period. Capacity to significantly predict outcome within 2 weeks of treatment was successful, based on data derived in the componential trial. How that was done and its implications for shortening clinical trials generally, is the subject of the next chapter. The conclusion from this chapter is that although either model is effective in achieving the primary aim of determining efficacy, the component-specific model can provide the information on onset, timing, sequence and most important, the nature of drug-induced clinical actions, that the established disorder-specific clinical trial is incapable of accomplishing. From the standpoint of economy of effort in clinical research, this research tells us that for small, additional amounts provided to conduct more intensive assessment of specific drug-induced changes, additional expenses that may easily be covered through possible shortening of the trial process, the field stands to gain new knowledge of great importance to both basic and clinical research in the field of neuropsychopharmacology.

It is useful to note also that the results of clinical trials carried out in the componential manner can contribute generally, to the science of psychopathology, to furthering the uncovering of the nature of the mental disorders and to finding more effective ways of treating them.

Chapter 8
Prediction and Shortening the Clinical Trial: Further Advantages of the Component-Specific Model

One of the more recent advantages of the component-specific model is its effectiveness in identifying predictors of outcome in trials of new drugs. There is as is well known, much to be gained by the capacity to predict early, within the first two weeks of treatment, whether a new drug is likely to be effective in resolving a targeted mental disorder in a 6 to 8 week course of treatment. For example, early knowledge of likely outcome will shorten the trial for a patient who would ordinarily have to experience an additional 4 to 6 weeks on an ineffective treatment. For the investigators and the funding source there is significant saving of effort and great expense in not having to prolong the trial of an "ineffective "drug beyond a two week period. These savings that serve to markedly benefit the patient also can be redirected toward the testing of new, potentially more promising treatments and do away with wasteful time and procedures.

The whole process of new drug development and evaluation can be facilitated, hopefully accelerating the pace of science in this sphere.

The capacity to predict outcome from early response in clinical trials has now been examined across several independent and metaanalytic large sample studies with surprising success. These studies which rely primarily, if not exclusively on the Ham-D for early assessment result in highly adequate predictive capacity. In our own work my colleagues and I have further refined the process by intensifying the measurement of early drug-induced clinical actions leading to potentially even more refined predictive formulae.

It is useful to first summarize from established trials, the findings, confined to the use of the Ham-D as the evaluative method, results of which indicate how effective two weeks is as a base for predicting outcome at 6 weeks of treatment. In this respect as background, Posternak and Zimmerman (2005) found that more than 60 % of improvement that occurred on active medication (and on placebo) took place during the first two weeks of treatment. Stassen et al. (1997) studies included a range of established ADs and greater than 1,000 patients, showing onset of improvement occurring within this period for 77 % of cases. It also showed that on average, no more than 10 % of patients who did not show any improvement within the first three weeks would become treatment responders at outcome.

M.M. Katz, *Clinical Trials of Antidepressants*, SpringerBriefs in Psychology, DOI 10.1007/978-3-319-26464-6_8

Szegedi et al. (2009) reported results from 4 studies comparing mirtazapine with active comparators or placebo in inpatients and outpatients, totaling 6907 patients on the relationship of early improvement at 2 weeks to treatment outcome. They found "early improvement" (EI), i.e., $\geq$20 % decrease in Ham-D, to predict stable response and stable remission with high sensitivity and specificity (81 and 87 %, respectively). Negative predictive values (no EI predicts no clinical response), as in the Stassen et al. studies were much higher (range from 82 to 100 %) than positive predictive values (19–60 %). They concluded that EI with ADs can predict subsequent treatment outcome with high sensitivity in patients with MDD; high negative predictive values indicating little to no chance of stable response in patients at outcome.

Thus, it was quite clear even if the studies used only the Ham-D as a measure of overall severity as the sole predictor, that early onset, initially uncovered by more refined methodology, could reliably predict six week outcome by the end of two weeks of treatment.

We researched this issue further within the confines of our study in 2004 (Katz et al.), using the more intensive analysis of early actions afforded by the MV set of methods in our component-specific trial. We established significant relationships between improvement as early as one week with outcome and extended these early findings by identifying specific components of the disorder, in which early changes were significantly predictive of outcome. These analyses uncovered the following:

By the end of the first week changes on several components of the disorder, induced by desipramine (DMI) were associated with clinical response at 6 weeks. They include the dimension, depressed mood-retardation (DM-MR), and behavioral and mood facets, depressed mood, anxiety, and somatization. These associations were sustained at 2 weeks. A reduction in the severity dimension, DM-MR, was also associated with outcome for paroxetine but did not appear until the end of two weeks of treatment.

The sensitivity and specificity analyses reinforced these relationships. Status on the DM-MR severity dimension at one week predicted outcome for DMI, resulting in 0.90 sensitivity and 0.88 specificity. A combination of behavioral facets can be used for paroxetine, as well as the DM-MR dimension, to also achieve acceptable sensitivity and specificity at 2 weeks.

In our most recent paper on prediction in which we recommend shortening of the clinical trial (Katz et al. 2015) we describe how the data from the 2004 study was reanalyzed to test and confirm the 2 week predictive hypothesis. That study however, was limited by the size and representativeness of the sample so the result was a recommendation that a "prospective" study be conducted which would utilize a much larger, more diverse sample of MDD, assembled from outpatient settings where most patients are currently treated.

The evidence so far is very convincing, however, that conducting new trials in the currently established manner, in which assessment of change is only required at baseline and at outcome, is at the least, wasteful and expensive. Further, in view of what we have learned about the mechanisms of drug action during these past several decades, it is also very unwise. It is clear from the large patient and diverse patient sample studies of Stassen et al. (1997) and Szegedi et al. (2009) that early improvement as measured on the Ham-D alone is highly predictive of response at outcome. In our componential approach to the problem (Katz et al. 2004, 2015), our modestly sized patient sample showed that early 2 week changes in major aspects of the disorder, could significantly strengthen predictive capacity and identify the early behavioral changes that initiate the recovery response. These advances await confirmation in a prospective large patient sample study, one that would provide a definitive componential profile on the nature, timing and sequence of changes that characterize the actions of a new drug. We elaborate on this important issue in the paper that recommends the shortening of the established clinical trial (Katz et al. 2015).

In the final chapter, I summarize the issues and the reasons for effecting major changes in the design and methodology for conducting future clinical trials that have been put forth in this book.

But before that, it is important to note that under selective circumstances, it is possible to take advantage of new technology and to record all aspects of a clinical treatment trial on videotape. The "video clinical trial" has been a subject of much of our research over the past three decades and has a distinct set of advantages over the conventional procedure. Its design and evidence of its advantages are presented in the next chapter.

Chapter 9
The Video Clinical Trial

This chapter begins by outlining in Table 9.1 the advantages that can be provided when a procedure that videotapes all interview and assessment procedures at multiple centers over a six week trial makes it possible to have all recordings evaluated at one central site.

I note that the video procedure took many years to develop (Katz and Itil 1970; Katz et al. 1989; Katz et al. 2006). It meant designing a standardized brief status interview of current symptomatology to be administered across diverse depressed patients at prescribed time points, during and at the end of treatment, and constructing or adapting observational rating scales for the interviews that would encompass common symptoms. But the rating method would also be designed to take advantage of the distinctive behavioral aspects that could be studied by observers who were *not* involved in the actual interview, e.g., expressive, physical qualities of the patient, and add the potential benefits of being able to view "before" and "after" interviews, concurrently.

The interview procedure for measuring status and change of depressed state was very similar to that described by Endicott and Spitzer (1979) for the SADS change (SADS-C) method (see Appendix I). The rating methods for the interview, the Video Interview Behavioral Evaluation Scales (VIBES) (Katz and Itil 1970, 2006) combined conventional descriptors of mood, behavioral and cognitive aspects of the disorder with scales especially designed to measure physically expressive and social behaviors. These new scales were subjected to psychometric studies in a sample of 46 diverse depressed patients, generating sets of components and factors: Expressive, symptom and social behavior components, and a set of severity dimensions, social withdrawal-retardation, agitation-anxiety, hostility and depressed mood-cognitive impairment.

These sets and components are illustrated in Table 9.2.

The reliabilities of these measures are summarized in Katz et al. (2006) as is their sensitivity to drug-induced actions compared directly with the sensitivity of the Ham-D evaluations. These findings as reported showed (1) the components

© The Author(s) 2016
M.M. Katz, *Clinical Trials of Antidepressants*, SpringerBriefs in Psychology,
DOI 10.1007/978-3-319-26464-6_9

Table 9.1 Advantages of video trials

1	Utilization of videotaped standard interviews of patients during course of multicenter treatment trials provides capacity to centralize in one location, observational data and ratings collected from several research sites
2	Trained raters in one center can conduct observational ratings on patients from all research sites, thereby reducing cross-center and cross-rater variability, and eliminating a major source of error variance in multicenter studies
3	Provides observation of physically expressive behavior, a sensitive area of change, but difficult to measure when rater is directly involved in interview
4	Permits introducing additional outside observers to judge behavior, e.g., social scientists and movement experts who focus on social and expressive behavior
5	Rater's detachment from interview eliminates variance in ratings due to involvement as interviewer
6	Capacity to view "before" and "after" treatment interviews concurrently, eliminates observer's need to recall the state of the patient prior to treatment, thus, allows for the "jumping of time" and increased sensitivity to change
7	The video approach maintains an archive of the trial. allowing for interobserver tests of diagnostic reliability, and later, convenient retrieval of data if required, to explore or test new observations
8	Thus, video is especially useful in early clinical trials in which potential values of novel treatments are examined in patients by experienced clinicians, i.e., "early drug evaluations", for treatments that may or may not be recommended for later control trials

Table 9.2 Brief VIBES factors and severity dimensions[*]

VIBES components		
Expressive scales	*Symptom scales*	*Social behaviour*
Motor retardation	Depressed mood	Positive adaptation
Agitation	Anxiety	Irritability
Distressed exp	Somatization	Agitation
Bodily tension	Cognition	Distraction
Detached-indecisive	Hostility	Suspicious
	Apathy-confusion	Openness
		Nervous
		Verbal aggression

Severity dimensions
Social withdrawal-retardation
Agitation-anxiety
Hostility
Depressed mood-cognitive impairment

Reproduced with permission of publisher from Katz et al. (2006) Int'l J Neuropsychopharmacology 2006
[*]Based on factor analyses of VIBES interview and paired ratings of 46 depressed patients

to be reliable; (2) the VIBES to be more sensitive than the Ham-D in measuring efficacy; (3) the VIBES to be more informative in identifying discrete behavioral aspects of the disorder that are impacted by the drugs. The conclusions following comparison of two pharmacologically different antidepressant drugs was that desipramine (DMI), an SNRI, initially "stimulated", i.e., increased motor activity and decreased depressed mood, and paroxetine, an SSRI, initially, reduced overall severity and anxiety.

In its demonstrated superiority to the Ham-D in assessing efficacy of DMI, in identifying specific changes in physical expression, agitation and bodily tension, and in being comparably sensitive to the Ham-D in detailing onset of clinical changes in 7 days, the VIBES demonstrates the enhanced sensitivity of this procedure in detecting and identifying the nature of drug-induced early behavioral changes.

Thus, with the component-specific trial, the video based study has much to inform about drug based clinical actions toward expanding knowledge about neurobehavioral mechanisms in addition to signaling a new drug's potential if such exists, for application in the treatment of other mental disorders.

Note certain specific advantages over the conventional trial include: (1) It allows the detached observer to utilize physical cues of change, e.g., "distressed expression", not easily observable when the rater is involved in conducting the actual interview; (2) permits "jumping time", introducing the opportunity to view baseline and post-treatment interviews simultaneously, thus, eliminating the need for the rater to recall behavior observed in earlier interviews.

Special Application in Multicenter Trials and Proof-of-Concept Studies

This capacity can be especially useful in early examinations of potentially new drugs, i.e., pre-clinical trial screening of candidate drugs. (3) The method has special advantages in *the conduct of multicenter trials,* common to the procedure for evaluating all new putative treatment drugs. It is noted that from the standpoint of efficiency, once they are collected in a video trial, all videotapes can be observed and rated by clinical staff at one central location. The centralizing of ratings, i.e., the utilization of well-trained raters in one setting to evaluate changes in patients from several research sites eliminates cross-center variance among rater groups. That is a common and significant source of error in the conduct of the established trial. Thus, the reliability and sensitivity of ratings is significantly increased with a secondary gain of markedly, reducing the cost of maintaining trained raters at each site.

This procedure, the details of which are further presented in Table 9.2 and Appendix I, are not easy to initiate in a study since it requires informed consent of all patients to be video recorded. So it is not likely to become a routine class of clinical trial. Nevertheless, it is as noted, particularly useful in pre-clinical screening or in small studies particularly where patient consent is not difficult to achieve, and basic video equipment available. In view of its standardized and well described procedures, it is ready to be applied. It should be seriously considered for application in early proof-of-concept studies.

Chapter 10
Conclusions

This document begins by noting the extremely expensive aspects of the conventional clinical trial in evaluating new, putative antidepressants. It cites the slow pace at which revisions were introduced to the statistics and to modifications of the sole method of evaluation, in order to enhance the sensitivity of this 50 year old model. These revisions have added little over this time to its sensitivity resulting in further discouragement in the field and a very obvious slowdown in the utilization of the model during the past two to three decades. Despite more than one third of acutely ill patients still found unresponsive to established drugs and the continuing need for more rapidly acting agents, there has been a failure to come up with drugs with novel mechanisms. The recent work with ketamine is noteworthy and promising for this area (Sanacora and Schatzberg 2015) for example, but the slow pace and the great expense of conducting new trials has led to abandonment of this area of research by many of the major drug companies.

A basic source of this state of affairs has been some confusion about what the clinical trial actually represents as a study. In its current form it remains in view of its randomized sample, double-blind method and control sample design a sound scientific study aimed at providing an unbiased result as to the efficacy of an experimental drug. The FDA requirement that two positive trials demonstrate efficacy strengthens the soundness of the approach to evaluating new drugs. The trial is not, however, in the natural stream of science. It is essentially applied science, in the end result, solely aimed at determining whether a new, potentially antidepressant treatment is efficacious, i.e., can meet the criteria established by Food and Drug Administration (FDA) to qualify for "marketability" as a treatment.

It appears that once one gets beyond the optimal dosage and marketability issues, there is no further use to which the study can be put, i.e., no further information of a scientific nature, e.g., about the sequence and quality of clinical actions induced by the new drug can be extracted from the trial nor are there explicit plans in most cases, for further analysis. The reason is that it is known

© The Author(s) 2016
M.M. Katz, *Clinical Trials of Antidepressants*, SpringerBriefs in Psychology,
DOI 10.1007/978-3-319-26464-6_10

from prior studies that the Ham-D cannot provide reliable information on any of the aspects or components of the "major depressive disorder". The trial would have to include additional methods to assess these aspects, methods that rarely are part of the conventional clinical trial.

It is the main intention of this book to call attention to the fact that the clinical trial as conducted today is simply an efficacy study and not one designed to advance the science in this sphere. A basic scientific study would require a more explicit analysis of the quality of the disorder being targeted for treatment, the components that structure that disorder and methods designed to measure possible changes in those components, as a function of the new, proposed treatment. If the treatment turned out to be non-efficacious for that disorder, the study could by way of an analysis of the nature and sequence of changes brought about by the agent, provide a profile of information on behavioral and neurochemical changes which could advance understanding of the target disorder or the neurobehavioral mechanisms underlying the efficacy or non-efficacy of the new treatment agent. It could also potentially signal that the agent due to its effects on certain dimensions of the targeted disorder, can find applicability in the treatment of other disorders, a very important step in the development of new treatments for the array of mental disorders.

This is what the component-specific and the video models for clinical trials are designed to accomplish, what clinical investigators, have a right to expect from a well-conducted investigation of the actions of a new treatment agent. This in fact, raises the aims of the trial. In contrast to the conventional marketing study with its limited aim of assessing efficacy, the new models raise it to the level of an experiment, the results of which can contribute significantly to the science of psychopharmacology in this area.

It not only contributes to the science, but offers its sponsor, the developer of the new treatment, a wealth of new information on the capacity of the trial drug and ideas that can advance development, further justifying the great expense and effort that went into its conduct. No longer an excercise in applied research, the clinical trial becomes a potential step in facilitating the advance to finding new and more effective treatments for this major mental disorder.

Appendix I
Four Case Studies of Patients in Multivantage (MV) and Video Models of Clinical Trials: Instructions for Scoring MV Components and Dimensions and Video Measure Profiles

Here the data is presented on four patients. Each patient was diagnosed as "major mental disorder" and examined within clinical trial model studies in which the multivantaged model (MV) (including the Hamilton Depression scale) or the VIBES model, or both, were applied.

They illustrate the use of the new methods included in these models, how the methods are administered and how they are scored. The reader will note that the MV model includes established methods, already validated by their authors, so that further details on these methods can be obtained by turning to the references provided at the end of the text. Also presented are the manner in which the various methods are scored and then combined to attain the profile of component and dimensional scores, unique to the MV and VIBES models.

The case studies:

1. Patient No. 1: Middle-aged grey haired man, well dressed, diagnosed as moderately depressed outpatient, responding well to treatment with desipramine. Analysis illustrates VIBES model and VIBES Standard Interview for tracking course of changes.
2. Patient No. 2: A well-dressed nurse in her early forties with a history of being moderately, but consistently depressed for several years. The MV method is illustrated tracking her treatment course over a 6 week period, demonstrating significant change and improvement with treatment.
3. Patient No. 3: Forty year old man diagnosed as "unipolar" with longstanding history of depression. MV and Video models show very little change during course of treatment.
4. Patient No. 4: Woman in her late 50's to early 60's presents as "classic" very, severe depression, hospitalized several times over the years prior to the current hospital stay. Very poor long term prognosis but contrary to expectations she has a remarkable response to imipramine, beginning within two weeks of treatment. MV analysis tracking changes over four week treatment course is presented.

© The Author(s) 2016
M.M. Katz, *Clinical Trials of Antidepressants*, SpringerBriefs in Psychology,
DOI 10.1007/978-3-319-26464-6

Patient No. 1

Middle aged man, well dressed, diagnosed as moderately depressed. The Hamilton Depression Scale (21 item form) score at baseline was 18 and his CGI score of severity was 4, signifying moderate depression. This case illustrates the use of the video model (VIBES) and is described first because it includes a transcript of a specially designed standard interview which is administered at each timepoint of the treatment trial, i.e., at baseline 0, 7, 10, 13, 22, 33, 40 days of treatment. To illustrate the procedure, the patient's response to the interview questions are transcribed for both the baseline (0) and the outcome (day 40, at 6 weeks) interviews only. To ease reading the patients' responses at baseline are emboldened; the responses on day 40 (outcome) are italicized. In regard to the task exercises, task 2 is timed, and tapping speed is measured.

This patient showed some retardation in tapping at baseline, but was otherwise not impeded in carrying out tasks.

Abbreviated Version of VIBESStandard Interview Schedule and Task Oriented Exercises

A.   Standard Interview Schedule

"Now I would like to ask you some specific questions about how you are feeling. I would like you to answer these questions as fully and completely as possible…"

1. Let's begin with…how are you feeling today?…**OK (baseline)**. *Great (day 40)*
2. What brought you here?……, **To find a medication that helps**. *Depression*
3. How long feeling this way?…**15 years, more so the last 10**. *10 years*
4. Describe your mood lately….**Don't know, nothing has changed**. *Positive*
5. Do you often feel sad or blue?…**Most of the time**. *Not any more*
6. Currently have crying spells or feel like crying? **No, crying is not part of it**. *No*
7. Are you more irritable lately? **No** *No*
8. Feel anxious, tense or restless? **Some restlessness, anxious**. *No, I am very calm*
9. Time in the day when you feel worse? **First, getting up in the morning**. *No, not at all*
10. In past few nights, problems with sleep? **No, matter of fact, slept all day Saturday**. *OK*
11. Appetite lately? **OK. Hasn't changed, the same**. *OK*
12. Past few days, change in sex drive, behavior? **No, still down**. *No, my sex drive is normal*

13. Trouble with your heart or breathing? **Trouble breathing, but because of my asthma**. *No, just the asthma*
14. Now having trouble with stomach, bowels? **No, active bowel movements**. *No*
15. Other body symptoms, urination, heavy limbs? **No**. *No*
16. Current trouble concentrating, reading, talk? **No**. *No*
17. Change in clarity, speed of thinking, memory? **No**. *Memory seems a little lighter, normal*
18. Now bothered by persistent worry, fears, ideas? **No**. *No*
19. Sudden fears or panic, no reason; if, how often? **No**. *No. Just worry about health*
20. Afraid something terrible going to happen? **No**. *No*
21. Worry about losing your mind? **No**. *No. Not any more*
22. Heard voices or seen visions past few days? **No**. *No*
23. How currently getting along with people? **OK. Not a lot of interaction, but get along fine**. *Get along well with people*
24. Angry a lot of the time? **No**. *No*
25. Lose temper easily? **No**. *No*
26. Feel people talking about you, out to hurt you? **No**. *No*
27. Feel now that thoughts controlled by others? **No**. *No*
28. Past few days, planned, attempted taking life? **No**. *No*
29. Feel problem is punishment for sin, bad deeds? **No**. *No*
30. Now able to work to own + others satisfaction? **No**. *Yes*
31. Have hobbies or social activities you enjoy? **No**. *No*
32. Enjoy your life? **No**. *Yes*
33. Feel useful and valued as person? **No**. *Yes*
34. Feel helpless? **No**. *No*
35. What do you think about your future, hopeful? **No**. *Yes*
36. Anything to say I haven't mentioned? **No**. *No*

B. **Task Oriented Excercises**

Now I would like you to do some tasks.

1. Subtract 3 from 20 and then 3 from the total. Continue until zero (time serial 3's task)
2. Would you smile for me?
3. Tap on table 30 X as fast as you can (time task)
4. Use your posture to show how you feel. (mood)
5. Copy the graph lines on the board behind you.

VIBES Profile

Factor measures				Interview sessions	
Score range: 4 (not at all) to 28(extremely)				Treatment	
Expressive scales	Baseline	2 weeks	5 weeks	6 weeks	Change[a]
Motor retardation	12.6	12.6	11.2	8.1	−4.5
Agitation	12.9	14.4	12.6	12.6	−0.3
Distr expression	12.3	7	7	7	−5.3
Bodily tension	16.3	16.3	14	14	−2.3
Detached-indecis	11.7	9.3	7	7	−4.7
Symptom scales					
Depressed mood	14	11	9	7	−7
Hostility	8.4	8.4	8.4	8.4	0
Anxiety	11.7	9.32	7	7	−4.7
Somatization	8.8	15.8	12.3	8.8	0
Cogn impairment	9.3	7	7	7	−2.3
Apathy-confusion	7	7	7	7	0
Severity dimensions (Range)					
Social Wd-Retard	11.4	12.4	13	18.6	7.2
Agitation-anxiety	35.5	33.7	27.6	27.6	−7.9
Hostility	17.4	17.4	17.4	17.4	0
Depr Mood-Cog Ump	23.3	18	16	14	−9.3
Social behavior scales					
Range: 4 (almost never)-28 (always)					
Positive adaptation	12	13	13	15	+3[b]
Anxiety	8	6	4	4	−4
Agitation	4	4	4	4	0
Irritability	5	5	5	4	−1
Distraction	5	4	4	4	−1
Suspicious	6	6	5	5	−1
Openness	11.2	12	11.2	12	8[b]
Verbal aggression	4	4	4	4	0
CGI(severity)	4	3	3	1	−3
CGI (improvement)	–	3	2	1	
Hamilton-D	18	17	7	5	−13

[a]Change: measured from baseline value to outcome at 6 weeks.
[b]To interpret, reverse scoring.

Case Summary

The profile at admission shows this man on the CGI scale of severity and the Hamilton Scale to be "moderately depressed".

The standard interview at baseline shows the profile of psychopathology and social behavior to be relatively high on anxiety reflected in mood and physical expression of tension (VIBES) and in depressed mood, with hostility not a major feature and social adaptation and behavior within normal limits. The response to treatment begins in week 2 with minimal improvement in overall severity focused mainly on reduction of depressed mood and minor change in anxiety level. By week 5 there is marked reduction in overall severity (Ham-D) depressed mood, indecisiveness and anxiety as patient demonstrates significant improvement over-all (CGI and components) as he progresses toward full response and as the final interview shows, clear recovery at outcome.

This picture of the patient's state at admission and the changes in components of the disorder that occur during the course of treatment, is based solely on the VIBES model of analysis. It illustrates the sensitivity of the VIBES in identifying specific changes induced by treatment. It matches, although not identically, the results of the more detailed MV method, that arrives at roughly the same results.

Patient No. 2

This man appears physically healthy, early forties in age, diagnosed as unipolar, markedly depressed with longstanding disorder at admission. The Hamilton at baseline was 24 and the CGI severity rating was 7, "extremely ill". This case is used to demonstrate the MV method but unlike the first patient, this patient shows minimal change and improvement at outcome of treatment with a significant increase in physical expression of the disorder.

Ratings were not available for certain of the interviews.

MV Profile Range

Components	Baseline	2 weeks	6 weeks	Change*
Depressed mood	6.05	4.69	4.85	−1.20
Anxiety	5.16	3.21	−	−
Retardation	3.92	−	1.64	−2.28
Agitation	2.53	−	3.10	+0.57
Hostility	4.63	3.68	1.37	−3.26
Somatization	2.29	1.64	8.3	+6.01

Components	Baseline	2 weeks	6 weeks	Change*
Distr expression	1.66	3.33	6.98	+5.32
Interp sensitivity	5.63	–	4.72	−0.91
Pos adaptation	2.78	–	7.6	+4.82**
Cogn impairment	1.94	1.19	5.0	+3.06
Slp disorder	0.75	1.33	2.8	+ 2.05
Dimensions				
				Change
Anx-Agit-Soma	4.98	–	–	
Depr Md-Retard	5.1	–	5.04	−0.06
Host-Int sens	3.6	2.87	2.95	−0.65
Ham-D (21 item)	31	26	22	−9.00
CGI severity	7	7	7	0
CGI Improvement	–	4	3	(minimal impr)

*Change: Measured from baseline value to outcome at 6 weeks.
**To interpret, reverse scoring.

Case Summary (Patient 2)

The baseline profile of pathology shows this patient to be significantly depressed in mood with equally high anxiety and hostile feelings, motoric retardation and relatively low scores on somatic complaints and cognitive impairment. At the end of treatment the patient is shown to have minimal improvement in motor retardation, feelings of hostility and social behavior. Increasing physical problems, however, are expressed in somatic complaints and physical expression of the disorder, with little to no change in overall severity and in major components of depressed mood and anxiety.

Patient No. 3

This patient is a nurse in her early forties, well dressed at admission, and diagnosed as moderately severe depression, longstanding in nature. The baseline Hamilton score is 18 and the GAS rating of social adjustment at 57. She illustrates a case assessed with the MV that responds well with early improvement in several aspects of the disorder at two weeks of treatment and progressive decrease of severity through to outcome.

MV Profile (Range 0–10)

Components	Baseline	2 weeks	6 weeks	Change*
Depr mood	3.13	2.39	1.53	−1.60
Anxiety	1.81	0.28	0.28	−1.53
Retardation	1.25	0.83	0.56	−0.69
Agitation	0.28	0.37	0.28	0.00
Hostility	0.76	0.69	0.56	−0.20
Somatization	2.51	1.74	0.98	−1.53
Distr expression	1.67	0.00	0.00	−1.67
Interp sensitivity	1.77	1.77	1.88	+0.11
Posit adaptation	3.58	5.13	7.99	+4.41**
Cogn impairment	0.76	0.00	0.00	−0.76
Sleep disorder	0.56	0.56	1.67	+1.11
Dimensions				
Anx-Agit-Somat	6.48	2.95	3.21	−3.27
Depr Md-Retard	4.38	3.22	1.09	−3.29
Host-Int Sensitiv	2.53	1.77	2.44	−0.09
Ham-D (21 item)	18	7	2	−16
CGI: Severity	4	3	1	−3
CGI: Improvement	–	3	1	

*Change: Measured from baseline value to outcome a 6 weeks.

**To interpret, reverse scoring.

| CGI[a] | | | Ret Mvmt | Agitation | DistrExpr |
Day	Sev	Impr	(SCOREA1)	(SCOREA2)	(SCOREA3)
0	4	–	1.33	1.17	1.25
3	4	5	1.50	1.00	1.50
7	4	3	1.33	1.17	1.25
11	3	3	1.33	1.17	1.50
14	3	3	**1.17**	1.33	1.25
17	3	3	1.33	1.17	1.00
21	3	3	1.33	1.00	1.25
28	1	1	1.00	1.17	1.00
35	1	1	1.00	1.00	1.00
42	1	1	1.17	1.00	1.00

[a]CGI: *Sev* severity, *Impr* improvement

Body dis	Dep Md	Hos	Anx	Soma	CogImp	Apathy
0	2.00	1.75	1.67	2.67	1.75	1.00
3	1.67	1.75	1.33	2.00	1.75	1.33
7	1.67	1.75	1.00	1.33	1.50	1.00
11	1.67	1.25	1.67	2.00	1.50	1.00
14	2.33	1.75	1.00	1.33	1.50	1.00
17	2.00	1.75	1.00	1.33	1.25	1.00
21	2.00	1.50	1.00	1.00	1.00	1.00
26	1.33	1.00	1.00	1.00	1.25	1.00
35	1.33	1.00	1.00	1.00	1.25	1.00
42	1.33	1.00	1.00	1.00	1.00	1.00

sd	Global rating	Rating of Change		SCOREA1	SCOREA2	SCOREA3	SCOREA4	SCOREA5	SCOREA6	scoreb1	scoreb2	scoreb3	scoreb4	scoreb5	scoreb6
1	0	4	10	1.33	1.17	1.25	1.67	2.00	1.00	1.75	1.67	2.67	1.75	1.00	1.00
2011	42	1	1	1.17	1.00	1.00	1.33	1.33	1.00	1.00	1.00	1.00	1.00	1.00	1.00

Case Summary (Patient 3)

This patient, moderately depressed at admission but with a longstanding disorder, presents a profile of pathology which is initially high on mood and somatic symptoms but lower on hostility and physical expression of the disorder. She shows relatively rapid response to treatment with desipramine, with significant decreases in two weeks in depressed mood and somatic complaints and improved social behavior as part of a marked early reduction in overall severity of the disorder. The recovery at outcome proceeds as predicted by the very significant "early improvement".

The case illustrates the drug's actions on components and the potential power of the two week response as a predictor of outcome response.

Patient No. 4

This patient, a woman of 60 years, represents a classically, severe depressive disorder, hospitalized at the time for treatment after several years of ineffective treatment. She was maintained for two weeks on placebo, then treated with imipramine, a dosage course that was gradually increased during the first week to 250 mg daily. She was then, maintained for an additional three weeks for 4 weeks of treatment. The patient represents an example of the remarkable effect that the tricyclics had early in its trials, on some patients who appeared to have the most intractable form of the disorder.

For practical reasons it was not possible to retrieve all of the MV method data from this study conducted in 1970, but there is sufficient data to illustrate the remarkable change that accompanied treatment during the period of 4 weeks in a patient that had not shown any change in illness status for several years.

MV Profile (Range 0–10)

Components	Baseline	2 weeks	3 weeks	4 weeks	Change[a]
Depressed mood	5.37	4.45	1.85	1.92	−3.45
Anxiety	3.21	4.35	2.18	2.32	−0.89
Retardation	4.12	3.91	2.33	2.03	−2.09
Agitation	0.97	2.29	1.15	0.89	−0.08
Hostility	0.33	1.38	0.55	0.50	0.17
Somatization	1.82	3.92	1.76	1.96	0.14
Distr expression	4.16	0.83	0.00	0.00	−4.16
Interp sensitivity	1.60	1.11	0.94	0.97	−0.63

Components	Baseline	2 weeks	3 weeks	4 weeks	Change[a]
Pos adaptation[b]	4.17	4.31	6.12	6.67	2.50
Cogn impairment	1.39	1.75	1.38	0.85	−0.54
Slp disorder	2.00[c]	3.08	2.58	1.83	−0.17
Dimensions					
Anx-Agit-Soma	4.00	6.82	3.84	3.50	−0.50
Depress Md-Ret	9.49	8.36	4.18	3.94	−5.55
Host-Int Sens	1.93	2.49	2.09	1.47	−0.46

[a]Change was measured by subtracting baseline value from week 4 value
[b]To interpret, Reverse scoring
[c]Prorated score

Case Summary (Patient 4)

This patient was severely and chronically depressed for years as reflected in baseline values on somatization, physical expression of the disorder and in the levels of depressed mood, anxiety and motor retardation reflected at the start of treatment. After 2 weeks of treatment we can see signs in her physical expression of a rapid response to treatment. Despite the still highs in depressed mood, anxiety and somatic complaints there are significant reductions in physical expression of the depressed mood. By the third week, there are marked reductions in depressed mood and anxiety with significant improvement in social behavior, hostility and motor activity. The patient, who had shown little change during a chronic illness lasting several years, is apparently well on her way to recovery by the end of the third week and this positive profile is maintained at outcome. The standard interviews at baseline and at outcome recorded on video provide an excellent display of the marked changes in clinical state. Her appearance and social poise at the outcome interview led to remarks by several of the raters that this patient "looked many years younger" than when they first interviewed her 4 weeks earlier.

Appendix II
Operational Definitions of State Constructs and Global Outcome Measures

These construct definitions are "operational", i.e., they are based on the factor measures that have been generated to define them. The factors that comprise the construct measures are listed in Appendix III.

	Factors
State Constructs	
Depressed Mood: A central mood that is expressed through feelings of sadness, downheartedness, worthlessness, loneliness and an inability to enjoy anything. The construct as defined, does not extend beyond the mood element of the depressive disorder	2
Anxiety: A mood and somatic state characterized by manifestations of fear, apprehension, severe tension bordering on panic; the subject uses such terms to describe the state, with evidence of both psychic and autonomic components	2
Retardation of Movement and Speech: A slowing down of motor movement, reactivity, and speech reflecting a reduction of available energy or of retardation of central nervous system functioning, generally	2
Agitation: Physical and mental restlessness which is expressed by the level and type of motor activity, with associated signs of hyperactivity, nervousness and irritability	1
Hostiity: The entire range of hostile affect and behavior from covert, "felt" anger and resentment to outward expressions of irritability, of threatening and other verbally aggressive behavior	2
Somatization: The extent to which psychopathology is expressed through physical symptoms. A range of symptoms usually or potentially reflective of anxiety and depression which can involve any or all of the systems of the organism	1
Distressed Expression: The extent to which emotional distress is manifested overtly in facial expression with such signs as tearfulness, sagging of the mouth, eyebrows drawn	1
Interpersonal Sensitivity and Suspiciousness: Extends from self-consciousness and minor sensitivity to criticism, to suspiciousness of the motives of others and "ideas of reference". Thus, shyness and "feelings easily hurt" would characterize one with a moderate amount of this affect, while high scores would signify strong paranoid tendencies	1

© The Author(s) 2016
M.M. Katz, *Clinical Trials of Antidepressants*, SpringerBriefs in Psychology,
DOI 10.1007/978-3-319-26464-6

	Factors
Positive Adaptation: Reflects generally positive affect and effective social behavior. Indicates extent to which there is good feeling within self, friendliness; comfortable, assertive, open behavior with others	2
Cognitive Impairment: Extent to which judgment, concentration, memory and thinking generally, are impaired; from minimum disturbance to the degree that there is actual confusion and psychotic impairment	2
Sleep Disorder: The extent to which the normal sleep pattern is disturbed, as manifested by early, middle or late insomnia, early awakening, difficulty falling asleep and apparent troubled sleep	1
Global Measures of Severity and Treatment Outcome	
Global Improvement: The extent to which the subject improves overall during the course of treatment (marked reduction of symptoms, generally over time) as judged by doctor (or trained rater) and from subject's report of symptom distress at end of the treatment period	1
Depressed State: This is a general measure of the severity syndrome. It takes into account all of the major characteristics of the depressive disorder, i.e., subjective state, activity level, appearance, and somatic symptoms; assesses the extent to which the "depressed state" is present	2

Appendix III
Composition and Scoring of Constructs, Dimensions and Overall Severity Measures

The constructs and dimensions are measured in patients through administration of a set of established psychological methods selected to assess the various behavioral, mood, cognitive and somatic aspects of the state of depression. For operational definitions of each of the 11 constructs and Global Outcome Measures see Appendix II. Further details are in Katz et al. (1984, 2004).

The methods that comprise the Brief MV battery are the following:

Observational Rating Methods

Schedule for Affective Disorders and Schizophrenia-Change Form (Endicott and Spitzer 1978)
Hamilton Depression Rating Scale (1960)
Clinical Global Impression (Improvement) (CGI) (Guy 1976)
Video Interview Behavior Evaluation Scales (Katz and Itil 1970)
NIMH Mood Scales (Raskin et al. 1969)
Ching K-S Social Behavior Scale (Sanborn and Katz 1977)

Self-Report Scales

Symptom Checklist 90 (SCL-90) (Derogatis et al. 1974)
NIMH Mood Scale (Raskin et al. 1969)

© The Author(s) 2016
M.M. Katz, *Clinical Trials of Antidepressants*, SpringerBriefs in Psychology,
DOI 10.1007/978-3-319-26464-6

Psychomotor Performance

Reaction time
Tapping Speed

There are 11 **Constructs** to describe the depressed state. Each is measured by the summing of factors from the various methods administered to patients diagnosed as "major depressive disorder". Three of the five overall severity scores listed are **dimensions**, measured by summing the factors most highly loaded on each, originally derived from a principal components analysis of the intercorrelations of the 11 constructs. The fourth severity measure is the total score on the 21 item Hamilton Depression Scale, the fifth, the Clinical Global Impression (CGI) (Improvement).

Measuring the 11 Constructs: The Composition of each of the Constructs. The Construct score is the sum of the items and factors, weighted equally, that are listed below under the source of the data.

Depressed Mood

Based on observer's (doctor or trained rater) rating of the severity of the mood from interview observations and the direct self-report of the patient.

1. **Interview Behavior**

SADS-C depression (i)*
VIBES Depressed Mood
Ham-D Depressed Mood (i)

2. **Subjective State**

SCL-90 Depression (Factor 5)**
NIMH Mood Depression (factor)

Anxiety

1. **Interview Behavior**

SADS-C Anxiety (i)
VIBES Anxiety (f)
Ham-D Anxiety-psychic (i)

2. **Subjective State**

SCL-90 Anxiety (f)
NIMH Mood Anxiety (f)

Retardation of Movement and Speech

1. Interview Behavior

SADS-C Psychomotor retardation (i)
Ham-D Retardation (i)
VIBES Retarded Movement and Speech (f)

2. Psychomotor Performance

Tapping speed
Reaction Time

Agitation

1. Interview Behavior

SADS-C Agitation (i)
VIBES Agitation (f)

Hostility

1. Subjective State

SCL-90 Anger, Hostility (f)
NIMH Mood Hostility (f)

2. Interview Behavior

SADS-C Subjective anger, Irritability (i)
NIMH Mood Hostility (f)

3. Somatization (comprised of symptoms as they are reported through doctor interviews and self-reports)

SADS-C Somatic symptoms (i)
Ham-D Somatic anxiety, gastrointestinal, hypochondriasis (i's)
VIBES Somatization (f)VIBES Bodily discomfort (f)SCL-90 Somatization (f)

Distressed Expression

1. Interview Behavior

VIBES Facial expression (f)
VIBES Guarded, Grandiose Thinking (f)

Interpersonal Sensitivity

1. Subjective State

SCL-90 Interpersonal Sensitivity
SCL-90 Paranoid (f)

2. Positive Adaptation

Subjective State
NIMH Mood Carefree (f)
NIMH Mood Friendly (f)

Cognitive Impairment

1. Interview Behavior

VIBES Apathy, confusion (f)

2. Subjective State

VIBES Cognitive impairment (f)
NIMH Mood Cognitive loss (f)
VIBES Insomnia (f)

Sleep Disorder

1. Interview Behavior and Subjective State

SADS-C Insomnia (early and late) (i)
Ham-D Insomnia (early and late) (i)
SCL-90 Sleep disturbance (f)

Dimensions

1. Anxiety-Agitation-Somatization-Sleep Disorder

The four construct scores that comprise this dimension are summed***.

2. Depressed Mood-Retardation of Movement and speech

The two construct scores are summed.

3. Hostility-Interpersonal sensitivity

The two construct scores are summed.

Overall Severity Scores

Hamilton Depression Scale Total (21 item)

CGI (improvement)

Depressed state

*i: test item

**To examine items comprising each test factor in the factorial methods, see basic reference on the method, e.g., for SCL-90, see Derogatis et al (1974).

*** The score for this dimension is divided by two in order to weight the score equally across dimensions.

Appendix IV
MV Methods for Measuring Constructs and Outcome Dimensions, Brief Version for Outpatient Studies

I. *Clinical rating methods*	*Average time to administer**	
Live SAD-C Interview + Ratings	Total: 40″	
1. Hamilton rating scale	10″	
2. SADS-Change Scale (SADS-C)	15″	
3. Video Int Behav Eval (VIBES)VIBES	10″	
4. Clin Global Improvement (CGI)		
5. Global Adjustment Scale (GAS)		
6. NIMH Mood	5"	
II. *Patient testing*	*Baseline, Outcome only*	*Interim/Brief Form*
Self-report scales	20″	
1. Symptom Checklist (SCL-90)	15″	SCL-60 10″
2. NIMH Mood Scale	10″	NIMH Mood-30 5″
III. Video interview ratings		Total 20–30″*
1. VIBES		
2. Ching K-S Social Behavior Scale		

*Ratings are mainly completed during course of interview

© The Author(s) 2016
M.M. Katz, *Clinical Trials of Antidepressants*, SpringerBriefs in Psychology,
DOI 10.1007/978-3-319-26464-6

References

Bech P (2011) Clinical psychometrics. Wiley, New York

Beck AT (1972) Depression: causes and treatment. University of Pennsylvania Press, Philadelphia

Collegium Internationale Neuro-Psychopharmacologicum (CINP) (2001)

Cuthbert BN, Insel T (2010) The data of diagnosis. New approaches to psychiatric classification. Psychiatry 73:311–4

Cuthbert BN, Insel T (2010) Toward new approaches to psychotic disorders. The NIMH research domain criteria project. Schizophr Bull 36:1061–2

Delgado PL (2000) Depression: the case for monoamine deficiency. J Clin Psychiatry 61(Suppl. 6):7–11

Derogatis LR, Lipman R, Rickels K, Uhlenhjuth EH, Covi L (1974) The Hopkins symptom checklist (HSCL): a measure of primary symptom dimensions. In Pichot P (ed) Psychological measurements in psychopharmacology: modern problems in pharmacopsychiatry, vol 7, pp 79–110. S. Karger, Basel.

DSM-5 (2014) American Psychiatric Association, Arlington

Dunbar GC, Fuell DL (1992) The anti-anxiety and anti-agitation effects of paroxetine treated depressed patients. Int Clin Psychopharmaocology 6:81–90

Endicott J, Spitzer RK (1978) A diagnostic interview: the schedule for affective disorders and schizophrenia. Arch Gen Psychiatry 35:837–844

Fixing the drug pipeline (2004) Economist 370:37–38

Gibbons RD, Clark DC, Kupfer DJ (1993) Exactly what does the Hamilton depression scale measure? J Psychiatr Res 27:259–273

Grinker R, Miller J, Sabshin M et al (1961) The phenomena of depression. Hoeber, New York

Guy W (1976) Early clinical drug evaluation program (CDEU) assessment manual of psychopharmacology. Department of Health, Education and Welfare, Rockville

Hamilton M (1960) A rating scale for depression. J Neurol, Neurosurg, Psychiatry 23:56–62

Hotelling H (1933) Analysis of statistical variables into principal components. JEP 24:417–441

Joyce PR, Mulder RT, Luty SE, McKenzie JM, Rae AM (2003) A differential response to nortryptiline and fluoxetine in melancholic depression: the importance of age and gender. Acta Psychiatr Scand 108:20–23

Kahn RJ, McNair DM, Lipman R, Covi L, Rickels K, Downey R, Fisher S, Frankenthaler LM (1979) Imipramine and chlordiazapoxide in depression and anxiety disorders: Efficacy in anxious outpatients. Arch Gen Psychiatry 43:79–85

Katz MM, Itil TM (1974) Video methodology for research in psychopathology and psychoharmacology. Arch Gen Psychiatry 31:204–210

© The Author(s) 2016
M.M. Katz, *Clinical Trials of Antidepressants*, SpringerBriefs in Psychology,
DOI 10.1007/978-3-319-26464-6

Katz MM, Robins E, Croughan J, Secunda S, Swann A (1982) Behavioral measurement and drug response characteristics of unipolar and bipolar depression. Psychol Med 12:25–36

Katz MM, Koslow S, Berman N, Secunda S, Maas JW, Casper R, Kocsis J, Stokes P (1984) Multivantaged approach in the measurement of behavioral and affect states for clinical and psychobiological research. Psychol Rep 55:619–791 (Monogr. Suppl. 1-V55)

Katz MM, Koslow SH, Maas JW, Frazer A, Bowden CL, Casper R, Croughan J, Kocsis J, Redmond E (1987) The timing, specificity, and clinical prediction of tricyclic drug effects in depression. Psychol Med 17:297–309

Katz MM, Wetzler S, Koslow SH, Secunda S (1989) Video methodology in the study of psychopathology and treatment of depression. Psychiatr Ann 19:372–381

Katz MM, Maas JW (1994) Psychopharmacology and the etiology of psychopathologic states: are we looking in the right way? Neuropsychopharmacology 10:139–144

Katz MM, Maas JW, Frazer A, Koslow S, Bowden CL, Berman N, Swann A, Stokes PE (1994) Drug-induced actions on brain neurotransmitter systems and change in the behaviors and emotions of depressed patients. Neuropsychopharmacology 11:89–1002

Katz MM, Tekell J, Bowden CL, Brannan S, Hoston JP, Berman N, Frazer A (2004) Onset and early behavioral effects of pharmacologically different antidepressants and placebo in depression. Neuropsychopharmacology 29:566–579

Katz MM, Houston JP, Brannan S, Bowden CL, Berman N, Swann A, Frazer A (2004) A multivantaged behavioral method for measuring onset and sequence of the clinical actions of antidepressants. Int J Neuropsychopharmacol 7:471–479

Katz MM, Houston JP, Brannan S, Tekell J, Berman N, Bowden CL, Frazer A (2006) A video method for the evaluation of antidepressant clinical and behavioural actions. Int J Neuropsychopharmacol 9:327–336

Katz MM, Berman N, Bowden CL, Frazer A (2011) The componential approach enhances the effectiveness of 2-week trials of new antidepressants. J Clin Psychopharmacol 31:253

Katz MM (2013) Depression and drugs: the neurobehavioral structure of a psychological storm. Springer, New York

Katz MM, Berman N, Bowden CL, Frazer A (2015) Evidence for shortening the clinical trial of antidepressants and a proposed paradigm for such studies. J Clin Psychopharm 35:324–332

Kendell RE (1968) The classification of depressive illnesses. Oxford University Press, London

Kielholz P, Poldinger W (1968) Die behandlung endogener depressionen mit psychopharmaka. Dt Med Wschr 93:701–704

Kornstein SG, Schatzberg AF, Thase ME, Yonkers KA, McCullough JP, Keitner GI et al (2000) Gender differences in treatment response to sertraline versus imipramine in chronic depression. Am J Psychiatry 157:1445–1452

Kraemer HJC (2013) Discovering, comparing, and combining moderators of treatment on outcome after randomized clinical trials: a parametric approach. Stat Med 32:1964–1973

Kuhn R (1958) The treatment of depressive states with G22355 (imipramine hydrochloride). Am J Psychiatry 115:459–464

Laird NM, Ware JH (1982) Random effects model for longitudinal data. Biometrics 38:963–974

Machado-Vieira R, Luckinbaugh DA, Manji HK, Zarate CA (2008) Rapid onset of antidepressant action: a new paradigm in the research and treatment of major depressive disorder. J Clin Psychiatry 69:946–958

Maas JW, Koslow S, Davis J, Katz MM, Mendels J, Robins e, Stokes P, Bowden C (1980) Biological component of the NIMH-clinical research branch collaborative program on the psychobiology of depression. Psychol Med 10:759–776

Montgomery SA, Asberg M (1979) A new depression scale designed to be sensitive to change. Br J Psychiatry 134:382–389

Morilak D, Frazer A (2004) Antidepressant brain monoaminergic systems: a dimensional approach to understanding their effects in depression and anxiety disorders. Int J Neuropsychopharmacol 7:193–218

Nelson JC (1999) A review of the efficacy of serotonergic and noradrenergic reuptake inhibitors for treatment of major depression. Biol Psychiatry 46:1301–1308

Papakostas GI, Perlis RH, Scalia MJ (2006) A meta-analysis of early sustained response rates between antidepressants and placebo for the treatment of major depressive disorder. J Clin Psychopharmocol 26:56–60

Pollack MH, Zaninelli R, Goddard A, McCafferty JP, Bellew KM, Burnham DB, Iyenger MK (2001) Paroxetine in the treatment of generalized anxiety disorder: result of a placebo-controlled flexible-dosage trial. J Clin Psychiatry 62:3

Posternak MA, Zimmerman MD (2005) Is there a delay in the antidepressant effect? A meta-analysis. J Clin Psychiatry 66:148–158

Quitkin FM, Rabkin JG, Ross D, Stewart JW (1984) Identification of true drug response to anti-depressant. Arch Gen Psychiatry 41:782–786

Pollack MH, Zaninelli R, Goddard A et al (2001) Paroxetine in the treatment of generalized anxiety disorder: result of a placebo-controlled flexible-dosage trial. J Clin Psychiatry 62:3

Raskin A, Schulterbrand JG, Reatig N, McKeon JJ (1969) Replication of factors of psychopathology in interview, ward behavior and self-ratings of hospitalized depressives. J Nerv Mental Disord 13:31–41

Robinson D (2007) Antidepressant drugs: evidence for onset of therapeutic effect. Primary Psychiatry 14:21–23

Rosenthal JD, Kakera R, McIntyre RS (2015) Cognitive effects of antidepressants in major depressive disorders: a systematic review and meta-analysis of randomized clinical trials. Int J Neuropsychopharmacol 10:1093

Sanacora G, Schatzberg AF (2015) Ketamine: promising path or false prophecy in the development of novel therapeutics for mood disorders? Neuropsychopharmacology 40:259–267. doi: 10.1038/npp.2014.261 published online 22 October 2014

Sartorius N, Baghai TC, Baldwin DC, Barrett B, Brand B, Fleischhacker W, Goodwin G, Grunze H, Knapp M, Leonard BE, Lieberman J, Nakane Y (2007) Antidepressant medications and other treatments of depressive disorders: a CINP task force report based on a review of the evidence 10:S1

Spitzer RL, Williams JB (1983) Instruction manual for the structured clinical interview for DSM III (SCID), revision. Biometrics Research Department, State Psychiatric Institute, New York

Stassen HH, Angst J, Delini-Stula A (1993) Time course of improvement under antidepressant treatment: a survival—analytic approach. Eur Neuropsychopharmacol 3:127–135

Stassen HH, Angst J, Delini-Stula A (1996) Delayed onset of action of antidepressant drugs? Survey of recent results. Eur Psychiatry 12:166–176

Szegedi A, Jansen WT, van Wugenburg AP (2009) Early improvement in the first two weeks as predictors of treatment outcome in patients with major depressive disorder: a meta-analysis including 6,562 patients. J Clin Psychiatry 70:344–353

Taylor MJ, Freemantle N, Geddes JR, Bhagwagar Z (2006) Early onset of SSRI antidepressant action: systematic review and meta-analysis. Arch Gen Psychiatry 63:1217–1223

Wong DT, Horng JS, Bymaster KL, Hauser Molloy BB (1974) A selective inhibitor of serotonin uptake: Lilly 110140, 3(p-trifluoromethylphenoxyl)-N-methyl-3-phenylpropylamine. Life Sci 15:471–479

Index

A
Antidepressant clinical trials, 1, 8, 17
Anxiety, 2, 6–11, 17, 20, 21, 24, 28–30, 32,
    35, 37, 44–47, 49–51, 54
Anxiety-agitation-somatization, 10
Arousal, 11, 17, 29

B
Bech, 3
Behavioral components, 3, 7, 9, 15, 17, 23
Benzodiazepines, 2, 30
Biological markers, 7
Bodily tension, 37, 44

C
Centralized clinical ratings, 2, 3, 9, 20, 37
CINP, 13
Classic depression, 9, 41
Clinical global improvement (CGI), 23, 42,
    44–46, 48, 50, 53, 54, 59
Cognitive impairment, 10, 20, 35, 46, 52
Component-specific, 9, 13–15, 20, 22, 25,
    27–30, 32, 37, 40

D
Depressed mood-retardation, 10, 11, 24, 28,
    29, 32
Depressive disorders, 2, 3, 5, 7, 8, 10, 11, 14,
    18, 21, 22, 40, 49, 51, 52, 54
Desipramine, 19, 41, 49
Diagnostic-specific, 15, 17
Dimensions, 8, 10–12, 17–19, 24, 28, 32, 35,
    40, 46, 47, 50, 53, 54, 59

Distressed expression, 10, 37, 51
DSM-5, 11, 12
Dunbar, 2, 30

E
Economist, 13, 15
Endicott, 20, 35
Evidence-based finding, 18
Expressive behavioral analysis, 35, 36

F
FDA, 12, 39

G
Generalized anxiety disorder, 8
Grinker, 9, 14
Guy, 23, 53

H
Hamilton depression rating scale, 53
Healthy controls, 5, 17
5-HIAA, 6
Holistic, 22
Hostility, 10, 11, 17, 18, 20, 24,
    29, 35, 44–47, 49, 50, 55

I
Imipramine, 5, 6, 41, 49
Impulsive hostility, 6
Itil, 35, 53

© The Author(s) 2016   65
M.M. Katz, *Clinical Trials of Antidepressants*, SpringerBriefs in Psychology,
DOI 10.1007/978-3-319-26464-6

J
Jumping time, 37

K
Kendell, 9, 14
Kielholz, 29
Kuhn, 5

M
Maas, 6, 9, 14, 17
MHPG, 6
Monoaminergic systems, 1
Montgomery- Asberg Depression Rating
    scale(MADRS), 2, 6
Motor retardation, 7, 9, 28, 29, 44, 46, 50
Multicenter trials, 37
Multisite studies, 6
Multivantaged (MV), 12, 20–22, 32, 41,
    45–49, 53, 59

N
Nelson, 18
Neurobehavioral actions, 6
Neuropsychopharmacology, 13, 30
Neurotransmitters, 5, 7
NIMH collaborative study, 17
NIMH mood scale, 20, 53, 59
Norepinephrine, 5–7, 9, 29
Normal controls, 9

O
Observational rating, 3, 9, 17, 20, 35, 53
Onset, 14, 15, 18, 22–24, 27, 28, 30–32, 37
Opposed neurobehavioral states, 11
Outcome dimensions, 59
Overall severity, 2, 6, 8, 15, 17, 23, 32, 37, 45,
    46, 49, 54

P
Paroxetine, 19, 22–24, 27, 28, 32, 37
Pharmaceutical companies, 1
Phenomenology, 9
Placebo, 2, 13, 20, 22–24, 27, 28, 31, 32, 49
Posternak, Zimmerman, 6, 19, 31
Prediction, 32

Predictors of outcome, 31
Principal components analysis, 9, 54
Profile of drug actions, 8, 11, 24
Proof of concept, 53
Psychological methods, 20, 35, 53
Psychometric studies

Q
Quitkin, 18

R
RDoC, 11, 12
Rosenthal, 23
Rush, 3

S
SADS-C, 20, 35, 54, 55
SCID, 22
SCL-90, 20, 53–55, 59
Secondary aims, 27, 14, 15, 23, 24, 27–29
Self-reports, 17, 20, 53, 54, 59
Sensitivity analyses, 3, 32
Sequence of actions, 14, 17, 28, 29
Serotonin, 5–7, 9, 10, 30
Shortening the trial, 30
Specificity analysis, 32
Spitzer, 22, 35, 53
SSRIs, 2, 6–8, 18, 27, 30
Stassen, 6, 18, 19, 31–33
State constructs, 51
Symptomatology, 9, 14, 35
Szegedi, 6, 18, 32, 33

T
Task-oriented performance tests, 43
Trial models, 27, 41
Tricyclic antidepressants, 6, 7, 18, 19, 27, 29

V
VIBES, 20, 35–37, 41, 42, 44, 45, 54, 59
VIBES expressive factors, 48
VIBES factors, 54
VIBES standard interview, 42
Video clinical trial, 33